UNDERESTIMATED

AN AUTISM MIRACLE

J.B. Handley and
Jamison Handley

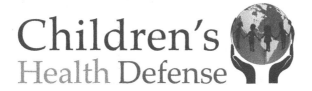

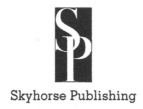

Skyhorse Publishing

Skyhorse Publishing books may be purchased in bulk at special discounts for sales promotion, corporate gifts, fund-raising, or educational purposes. Special editions can also be created to specifications. For details, contact the Special Sales Department, Skyhorse Publishing, 307 West 36th Street, 11th Floor, New York, NY 10018 or info@skyhorsepublishing.com.

Skyhorse® and Skyhorse Publishing® are registered trademarks of Skyhorse Publishing, Inc.®, a Delaware corporation.

Visit our website at www.skyhorsepublishing.com.

10 9 8 7 6 5 4 3 2

Library of Congress Cataloging-in-Publication Data is available on file.

Cover design by Yuneekpix

Print ISBN: 978-1-5107-6636-5
Ebook ISBN: 978-1-5107-6637-2

Printed in the United States of America

CONTENTS

*For EV, who never gave
up on any of us.*

Introduction

Sometimes real superheroes live in the hearts of
small children fighting big battles.

—Anonymous

Autism means different things to different people, which shouldn't be any surprise. The official term for autism is "Autism Spectrum Disorder," and that word *spectrum* ensures that people will forever be confused when trying to understand how the word autism serves to describe any one individual. That's why it's important to start right here in describing a very special young man with autism, my son Jamison Havener Handley, henceforth known in this book as "Jamie."

You can find an adult with autism, unable to talk, prone to raging, wearing a helmet to protect themselves from self-injury, unable to meet even basic daily needs, living in a full-care facility where the goal of care providers is simply to keep the person safe and alive. Another person with autism might be attending college, their differences subtle enough to escape the notice of most of their classmates. You might even say that autism has become fashionable. Jerry Seinfeld, before taking it back, told Brian Williams on NBC that "I think, on a very drawn-out scale, I think I'm on the spectrum." And what evidence did he have for his autism? "Basic social engagement is really a struggle,"

Mr. Seinfeld explained. If only that were the autism we've lived with for the past seventeen years.

My wife, Lisa, and I will sometimes say, really only to each other, that Jamie has the "real autism." At the risk of offending someone on the spectrum reading this book, please withhold judgment until I explain what that means for us. Jamie doesn't speak. When extremely frustrated, he can explode into a fit that ends in self-injury, the kind that's sent him to the emergency room. He has distinct mannerisms and will "stim" in a way that clearly signals to the onlooker that Jamie has a unique disability. He has compulsions that can be hard for him to manage, like tearing leaves into very small pieces. In school, it was clear to Jamie's teachers that he was kind, sensitive, and able to track and understand many of the things said and going on around him—what's known as "receptive language"—although how much he was tracking no one really knew. Communication has always been Jamie's biggest challenge. With the exception of a handful of words to get his basic needs met—phrases like "shower please," "go car," "help please"—Jamie has been a non-speaker his whole life, despite many different communication methods we and his teachers tried to help get him speaking. This inability to speak has not only made assessing Jamie's cognitive functioning and intelligence level nearly impossible, it has relegated him to a "life skills" class in a school here in Portland, Oregon, called Victory Academy, henceforth known as "Victory," that only serves children on the spectrum. What does it mean to be in a "life skills" class? In my opinion, it is a nice way of saying something to this effect: "We don't think you have the cognitive ability to take academic coursework, so we will focus on giving you the skills to be as independent as possible." As he's gotten older, Jamie's school days have increasingly been spent learning how to do laundry, clean up, use a debit card, cook, and master other basic tasks that will help him navigate his looming adulthood.

Jamie's teachers have always been quick to tell us how much they love Jamie's gentle, loving nature, his warmth, his kind presence, and his infectious joy on display during favored activities. But even the most optimistic evaluation of Jamie given by the same caregivers contorting themselves to not hurt our feelings always left me feeling depressed and worried, deeply worried, about Jamie's future. They couldn't really tell us much about Jamie's cognition. They didn't think he could read. Math? He could count to 100, but that appeared more rote. Processing a mathematical equation? He'd never shown he could. How do you plan a future around that type of guidance? We had no idea if Jamie had dreams, goals, or hopes for his adult years; it was all conjecture. Heck, did Jamie even know what dreams or goals *were*? I didn't know for sure, because we had no real sense of how Jamie was processing the world. Walking out of these painful progress reports, Lisa and I would be saddled with the same harrowing question that so many other parents of children with the "real autism" face: what will my child do when I'm gone?

My best friend in the world is Drew, and he lives in Salt Lake City. His two children are, by my standards, utterly perfect, and the challenges he faces as a dad are, compared to mine, pretty damn trivial. He knows this, and he does his best to understand what life is like for me. When he visits, he takes great pains to connect with Jamie, and I love him for his effort. For whatever reason, as I sat down to write this book, my mind kept returning to a conversation we had, several years ago. I was standing in the backyard, on my phone. Jamie, as is often the case, was between our bushes, shredding leaves, seemingly in his own world. As he usually does, Drew was asking me sincere questions about Jamie, trying to better understand how things were really going, like "No dude, how are you really?" I was trying to appear the optimist—find something positive to say about our plight and Jamie's dimming prospects for a future. I guess I wasn't ready to lose it on the phone with my best buddy. That's when I said something to Drew that I'll never, ever forget. "It may be a blessing in disguise: Jamie has the kind of autism where he doesn't even know he has autism. He's oblivious and happy, not self-conscious," I reasoned, "and in a sense, maybe we're blessed. If we can keep finding things that keep Jamie happy, he can still have a happy life, and what he doesn't know or understand can't hurt him."

Yes, I said all that. I believed what I said, too, I really did. And I couldn't have been more wrong. I mean, wrong by a trillion miles wrong. My own son. Thank God for that, thank God for Jamie, and thank God for the miracle that has made this book possible.

I

Twelve Months

1

Twelve Months

Vancouver Island

There is no darkness but ignorance.
                              —William Shakespeare

Some birthday we're having for Jamie. August 21st has become perhaps my least favorite day of the year. It's no longer a day where I celebrate Jamie's birthday, but rather a day that reminds me of all that's been taken from him and the life he has missed out on. This one hurts a little more. It's 2019, and Jamie is seventeen today. In twelve months, the state will consider Jamie an adult, which means Lisa and I must go through major legal bureaucracy to declare Jamie incompetent and become his legal guardians. Happy Birthday!

We're all in Canada now, on Vancouver Island to be more specific. When I say, "we," I mean my wife, Lisa, my twelve-year-old daughter, Quinny, and Jamie. We're a family of five, but Sam, our oldest, has just headed back to college for his sophomore year, and we've escaped Portland partly to help distract from Sam's departure, which has proven to be excruciating for all of us. We also have another reason to be here, and it involves the birthday boy.

The Trans-Canada Highway is spectacular as we leave the confines of the charming city of Victoria on our way up to the tiny town of Duncan in the mountains. It's early, and none of us are morning people. We wolf down breakfast at the hotel and, as always, are pressed for time. If you think our vacation sounds glamorous, this might change your mind: we're headed to a clinic to give Jamie the first of ten fecal microbial transplants, or "FMTs" as they are known in the natural health world. Recently, an Arizona State professor published a paper showing that FMTs were effective in lessening the symptoms of autism in a small trial of kids like Jamie, and we've decided to give it a try. Unfortunately, the FDA isn't allowing FMTs for autism yet in the US, but Canada allows them, so on "vacation" we've gone.

This isn't the first time we've tried something non-traditional to help Jamie's autism. There have been so many that I've long lost count. Luckily for me, Lisa has been an enthusiastic copilot in trying anything to help Jamie. In fact, Lisa has served the important role of scrutinizing any new idea I come across and doing her best to ensure that any new treatment (we call them "interventions") passes a simple test: it won't hurt Jamie or risk making things worse. Looking back, many of these interventions have benefited Jamie. Removing gluten from his diet really calmed him down. When we added methyl B-12 (a vitamin), Jamie regained a few words. Hyperbaric Oxygen Therapy (HBOT) seemed to have a noticeable impact on the health of his gut. Even today, we keep a very strict diet, and Jamie never eats gluten, dairy, soy, or any artificial colors, sweeteners, or preservatives. He rarely has sugar. And Jamie's body has responded. Physically, he's robustly healthy, he never gets sick, and he sleeps great. Neurologically? Things remain complicated, but Jamie has certainly regained the ability to sit and concentrate and focus on tasks. Like I said, it feels like everything has helped a little, but we're still miles from where we'd like to be, so we keep going.

Through networking with parents, talking to the clinic here in Canada, and reviewing the published science, we feel FMT is one of the more compelling interventions we've heard of, so our hopes are up as we motor north through the undulating, deep green hills of Vancouver Island. Lisa and Quinny drop us off at the clinic and head out for some sightseeing and shopping to pass the time. This is day one of ten, and Jamie and I will be here for a few hours. While I have no idea if he understands what's about to happen, I have taken great pains to explain everything to Jamie, and, as usual, he's proving to be a great sport. This is the same kid who sat with me patiently in the claustrophobic confines of a hyperbaric oxygen chamber for more than 100 "dives," so I'm hoping on some level he's used to it.

As we enter the clinic, I'm surprised to learn that Jamie is in fact the first person with autism they've ever treated. My guess was that after the Arizona State study, American parents would be beating the door down here in Canada. Far from it, they tell me, and I can see the concern on the faces of the clinicians as they work to navigate Jamie's unique disposition. You can tell when someone is used to being around people with autism, and they aren't. That dissipates quickly, because Jamie is incredibly compliant, while enduring both an enema and a scary-sounding but relatively benign rectal catheter. I'm overwhelmed sometimes when I think about what Jamie has endured, and this is one of these moments. Does he understand? Does he realize this might help him and that's why he's being so patient and amazing? These kinds of thoughts come often, and more and more lately as Jamie gets older. I'm often in awe of my son, really, because he's almost always in a good mood, he seems to find joy in the little things, and everyone who meets him notes his warmth, kindness, and calm presence. "What keeps him going?"

I wonder, "Where does he find the joy?" These thoughts always lead to the inevitable, and painful, longing to know what's going on inside Jamie's head. How does he see the world? What does he understand? As the years have passed, I've painfully resigned myself to never knowing, but whenever I let that thought bubble up, the pain is acute.

Most of the time in the clinic is spent waiting. I'm sitting by Jamie who is horizontal on a small bed, slightly inverted to give his recently received microbiome "transplant" the best chance of remaining in his bowels, hopefully replacing an unhealthy microbiome with a healthy one. It sounds simple, and it really is. Given our downtime, the clinician is peppering me with questions about Jamie. I'm always a little uncomfortable answering questions in Jamie's presence about him, it somehow feels wrong—he should be the one answering. And, what if he is tracking me? I don't want to offend him. The familiar questions about autism always leave me depressed, because questions inevitably lead to talk of the future. "What are Jamie's aspirations?" the clinician innocently asks me. I have no idea what Jamie's aspirations are. Does he even know what "aspirations" means? It's so challenging to try and glean what sort of life Jamie hopes for. Lisa and I constantly search for clues. He's very happy at the ocean. He likes swings, and he's always delighted when his big brother, Sam, comes back from college. That's not exactly a blueprint for the next sixty years, is it?

Sitting in this clinic also reminds me of the most dangerous drug for an autism parent: hope. I can feel it creeping in again. Maybe FMT will work for Jamie the way it worked for some of the kids in the study. Some of the reports include dramatic improvements. Reading the descriptions, many of the study participants sound similar to Jamie. Could this somehow make Jamie talk? I've learned to quickly suppress these optimistic hopes, because the hangover, the letdown when miracles don't happen, is usually how these things end. I remind myself that even a modest improvement is a good thing, and I distract my brain with the need to comfort Jamie as he lays there, patiently waiting for the timer on the wall to tick down and let us know the rest of our day on this beautiful island is free. We're all headed to the ocean.

Portland

Faith is the bird that feels the light
when the dawn is still dark.

—Rabindranath Tagore

"I just got the call," I tell Lisa as I jump into my car. It's October now, we're back into the familiar rhythm of two kids in school. What I haven't yet told her is that this one sounds worse than most, I won't really know for sure until I get there, so I won't burden her with the thoughts. "The call" is the inbound call from Tricia, the head of Jamie's school, Victory. She always tries to be calm, even reassuring, but I know that if I see her number light up my phone in the middle of a school day, it's bad news. Jamie has had another outburst, another succession of events that ends with Jamie hitting himself, very hard, on his head. He hits himself, usually with the back of his hand. It's awful.

When it happens at home, I can intervene. We know the signs, and I can usually get there before Jamie lands the first closed fist on either his forehead or his crown. Jamie's a big kid now—6'2" and 220 lbs—but, luckily, I'm a big guy, too, and I can restrain him until he calms down, until the overwhelming feeling to self-injure passes. It takes 5–10 minutes, and then Jamie snaps out of it. Afterward, he's always shaky, thirsty, and seems shocked, as if even he doesn't know what happened. A doctor tells us it's involuntary at some point, the brain just sort of takes over. The lead-up is always the same: he starts stomping, then jumping, then shaking his arms vigorously over his head, moaning loudly. We know the sounds, we know the signs. We sprint through the house to locate him, usually in time to ward off disaster. One time, we didn't make it, and one of the head hits caused the back of his hand to blow up like a balloon. I rushed him to the ER. Somehow, he didn't break it.

The drive to Victory passes through beautiful countryside. It's a solid thirty minutes from our house, although at my speed I'll get there sooner. The quiver in Tricia's voice leaves me very stressed and unsettled. She sounded grave. I often joke, darkly, that I don't have PTSD about Jamie because, well, there's nothing "post" about the trauma I endure; it still happens all the time. Of course, it's no joke and all, and I'm certain my nervous system is starting to feel the effects. States of anxiety seem to last longer lately. Like now, I know my day will pretty much be shot because my nervous system is redlining. Sleep is becoming a real challenge. I turned fifty a few months ago. How long can I endure?

I pull up to the school, leave my car in the turnaround, and race to find Jamie. As usual, he's outside. His teachers know nature calms him down. He's sitting quietly now. You wouldn't know anything has happened if not for the look on the face of his favorite teacher, Molly. She no longer teaches Jamie day to day, but whenever Jamie has an issue, she's the first one called. Molly is clearly shaken, and she's known Jamie since he was nine, so almost a decade now. "It was a rough one, J.B., I'm sorry to tell you," Molly starts, "the worst one I've seen." She's tearing up as she tells me. I know she loves Jamie. I also know how awful it is to watch a child hit himself on the head. "We counted at least a dozen hard hits to the head. Really hard." I'm tearing up, too.

There's a tiny silver lining in all this. It's actually the first explosion like this since we did FMT back in August, and this is kind of a miracle, because last school year, these outbursts were happening almost every week. My life had basically turned into one of waiting to get the call from Tricia to come get Jamie.

Lisa and I are constantly brainstorming to figure out why Jamie is having these outbursts at school. Home outbursts are comparatively rare, and when they happen, we usually can reconstruct a reason, something that made Jamie feel frustrated or anxious. At school, we're at the mercy of his well-intentioned teachers, and they aren't seeing a consistent pattern.

Unfortunately, in order to address the safety concern we all have for Jamie, many of his most enjoyable activities at school have been curtailed, because they risk setting him off. No more trips to the climbing gym. No more music class. No more running on the treadmill. At some point, each of these things has been a precursor event to Jamie's outbursts, so they're out. I've begun to wonder if Jamie even enjoys school anymore. Most mornings, as we approach the door, he starts driving his teeth into my shoulder, a habit he usually saves for times of stress. Is he trying to tell me something?

The ride home affirms another observation that's always true. As soon as Jamie's picked up after these incidents, he's perfectly fine. Giddy, in fact. It's a crisp fall day, but dry. I decide to take Jamie for a bike ride—we use a tandem. This is one of our favorite activities, and he seems to love it.

Lisa calls. She was on the opposite side of town and tied up when Tricia called, so she hasn't heard the news. I'm skilled at biking and talking, so I answer. Part of me would rather not tell her; I've already had to face and process the scale of self-injury today, so why burden her with it, too? That's not how we roll though—we are partners on this journey—so I share the bleak news about Jamie's self-injury, and the fact that this was the biggest one yet. Her tears come quickly, she feels Jamie's pain the way only a mother can.

As she talks, a feeling overtakes me. It's one that's been cropping up more often in the last year. I don't want to admit it, especially not to Lisa. I've always been her Superman, the family provider, the rock. But I'm fraying at the edges. While the FMT has calmed Jamie down and reduced the self-injury, we've seen no change in cognition, no words, no normalization of behaviors. Sure, it's early, it's been only about six weeks. But, and I can only say this to myself, I'm disappointed. Moreover, he's seventeen. Have we missed our window? Is Jamie simply who he is? I hate these thoughts. I try to will them out of my head, but they are hanging around more often, dragging me down. For the first time in this seventeen-year autism odyssey, I'm just not sure if I'll make it. I don't really know what that even means. I'm not suicidal, but the prospects of thirty or forty more years like this feel daunting. Really fucking daunting.

I reveal a sliver of this to Lisa. I tell her the magnitude of this outburst really scared me. I'm scared for Jamie. How could he not have a concussion from all this hitting? Even if this only happens every few months, how much can his brain endure? Should we take him out of school? Should he wear a helmet (which he would probably rip right off)? He seems so much happier at home. If he stays home, we know the number of incidents will go down, if not disappear. In moments like this, Lisa tends to find a way to rescue me. She reminds me that, every day, more progress is being made to discover how to help kids with autism. Jamie's still so young. Something's going to give, something's on the horizon.

I hear none of it. I just don't believe her today. The scared look in Molly's eyes, I'm feeling the magnitude of Jamie's self-harm. Things feel very dark. Hoping for a miracle feels foolish. I pedal harder, hoping the endorphins will calm my racing brain.

Oceanside

To love someone with all of your heart requires
reaching them where they are with the only
words they can understand.

—Shannon L. Alder

It's early December. I'm always grateful for the Oceanside Hustle, a lacrosse tournament here in Southern California held at this time every year, just as Oregon is turning into a dark, wet, depressing mess.

Sports has always been a refuge for our family. Lisa and I were both athletes, and our older son, Sam, came out of the womb looking for a ball to throw, a bike to ride, or a bat to swing. Through him, we became active participants in the club sports scene, and Sam's teams have taken us on weekend tournament trips too numerous to count. As Sam aged, he narrowed his focus, and lacrosse became his thing. His God-given athleticism and unique ability to practice nonstop made him a sought-after player by major college programs, and he ended up a University of Pennsylvania Quaker in the Ivy League.

But we're not in California for Sam; we're here for his twelve-year-old sister, Quinny, who is doing her best to walk in her older brother's footsteps. She has many of her brother's athletic gifts, and lacrosse has emerged as her favorite sport, too.

This is our sixth year in a row at this tournament, and we always rent the same house that sits right on the ocean. It's our nod to Jamie, who always seems happiest when near the water. It's also a nod to the fact that we always travel as a unit, no matter what. In Jamie's early years, this led to many stressful travel moments, but we endured them all, and at this point Jamie is a calm and enthusiastic traveler. A self-taught swimmer, Jamie will rush into the water no matter the temperature and loves getting bashed by waves. It sounds scary, but he's a remarkably competent waterman, so it's a joy anytime we find ourselves on a coastline.

It's Friday night, the tournament starts tomorrow, Quinny and Lisa are out at her team's dinner, and I'm home with Jamie. This is our most common configuration, and it feels like there are an infinite number of times where an event or invitation isn't Jamie-friendly, so I just opt to stay with him while Lisa and Quinny venture out.

The sun is quickly descending behind the Pacific's dark winter waters, but Jamie is undaunted, still playing in the Pacific. I'm standing at the water's edge, hoping I won't need to jump in for any reason, because the water is freezing. The truth is, I never have to, but I'm still on guard. These moments at the ocean's edge, with Jamie seemingly at his happiest, are always a time for reflection.

My beautiful baby boy, soon to be a man, frolics in his favorite place. Is there more to life than being happy? Is being happy with simple pleasures enough? With Jamie, I've started to accept that it might have to be. Can we construct a life for him that ensures enough simple pleasures to bring him consistent joy?

As darkness takes over the sky, to my surprise, Jamie comes out of the ocean without my prodding—even he must have a temperature minimum. Luckily for the both of us, this house has a hot tub, and we spend the next hour there defrosting. The house is perched extraclose to the ocean, and the pounding waves are all we can hear while floating in the hot water. It's a pretty divine moment, and I'm not shy about appealing to God at times like this. "Please God, give me the strength and stamina to give Jamie a life of joy and meaning, and please watch over him and always keep him safe."

These simple prayers, I still remember when they started. It was the first night, on our computer, when Lisa and I started exploring the word "autism." Jamie was only a toddler, maybe twenty months old, but he was starting to do odd things. There's this simple little test on the Internet called the M-CHAT where twenty quick questions, answered in less than five minutes, can change your whole life. He basically failed the test, which meant a near guarantee of autism. And that first night, after the failed M-CHAT, was the first night I ever prayed to God. I wasn't ready to believe the test result, so I viewed the prayer at the time as just a hedge. That was almost sixteen years ago.

As I sit in the hot tub, lost in thought and prayer, my relationship with the man upstairs is actually pretty strained. From my perspective, despite sixteen years of consistent appeals, we really haven't seen much. What I don't know floating there is that in two short weeks, everything is going to change.

And I mean everything.

Beaverton

*Faith is taking the first step even when you don't
see the whole staircase.*

—Martin Luther King, Jr.

It's December 9, 2019, and the part of living in Portland that's always been the toughest for me is in full swing: early darkness and dreary weather. It's only 5:20 p.m., but it's already pitch-black outside and I find myself sitting, uncomfortably, on the floor of a small gym as Quinny, soon to be thirteen, is hustling up and down the court with her club basketball team. My outings with Quinny aren't nearly as frequent as I'd like, but the moments when it's just she and I are always an oxygen break for me. She's considerate, loving, innocent, and sweet, and at the same time she's emerging as both an extremely fierce competitor and a seriously intelligent student. Her social life is always busy, and she finds a way to be kind to everyone. She makes me damn proud, and I'm staying to watch her whole practice, partially because this gym is on the other side of town, but really because I simply enjoy watching my baby girl from afar. With a little bit of space between us, I see more clearly the woman she's becoming, which always leaves me toggling between trepidation and joy.

A text chimes. I check my phone. I'm not sure what to think. Honey Rinicella lives in Philadelphia, and we've become what can best be described as autism pen pals. I don't hear from Honey often, but we share a passion for trying to get our sons better—her Vince is roughly the same age as Jamie—and we've shared ideas over the years for anything that might help our boys. "Hey, have you heard about this new light therapy? I have a friend who it helped." That kind of thing. This network of autism parents is quite vast, and most of the best ideas we've tried to help Jamie have come from other parents.

When my son Sam decided to go to college in Philadelphia, I reached out to Honey to let her know, and she was quick to offer to be there for Sam in a pinch. This is no surprise, Honey is known throughout the autism community for her willingness to help anyone, anytime. It's even more impressive because we've yet to meet each other in person. She also introduced her oldest daughter to Sam, and the two became friends—the bond of having a brother with autism will do that. Knowing what I do about Honey, I presume the text will be something she's stumbled across that might have some promise to help Jamie.

"Have you heard of Spelling to Communicate?" Honey writes. "No. What's up?" I quickly respond. "We're seeing crazy words out of Vince," she responds.

Context needed: Vince, her son, is just like Jamie. He doesn't talk. He has "mannerisms," which is the word we use to describe the unusual body movements and noises many on the spectrum make. He has the "real autism." No one says they are seeing "crazy words" out of Jamie or Vince, and I know Honey is a real autism parent who would never joke like that, so I read her text with what can only be described as intense confusion.

"Come again?" is all I can muster in my text. The next thing that arrives is a screenshot of what appears to be some sort of question-and-answer script, and it reads like this:

What do you think about Mr. Rogers' open heart, yet matter-of-fact delivery?

IT IS TOUGH TO STRIKE SUCH A DELICATE BALANCE. YOU NEED TO HAVE THE MESSAGE IN A CLEAR YET WARM DELIVERY. CHILDREN ARE SO SENSITIVE TO WORDS THAT THEY MUST BE CHOSEN WITH ALL THE CARE IN THE WORLD.

I don't know what's going on. I reread the screenshot. "WTF?" is my response. Honey quickly writes, "the words in all caps, that's VINCE." Nothing is clear to me, that seems impossible, I'm not sure where to even put that. Another screenshot appears. I'm equally bewildered:

Drennan used her disadvantage to her advantage. What are your thoughts on that mindset?

IT IS THE MINDSET OF DIFFERENCE MAKERS. TIME AFTER TIME, THESE PEOPLE CHOOSE TO SEE THE OPPORTUNITY INSTEAD OF THE OBSTACLE. THIS IS A LEARNED POINT OF VIEW. SOME HAVE THE INNATE ABILITY BUT IGNORE II. IT IS A SHAME.

"That's Vince?" I ask. I'm not believing this. I know Honey would never joke like this, but things really aren't adding up. She drops another screenshot on me:

Would you rather do something and not get the publicity, or would you rather receive the acknowledgment?

I'D RATHER NOT RECEIVE THE ACCOLADES. I'M GREAT WITH A LIFE IN SOLITUDE WITH MY PEOPLE. ACCOLADES AREN'T EVERYTHING. I'M CONTENT WITH MY ACHIEVEMENTS GOING UNRECOGNIZED. AS LONG AS THEY MAKE A POSITIVE IMPACT I AM HAPPY.

I get up from where I'm sitting in the gym and head for a quiet room off to the side, no longer aware of my surroundings. I'm in a state of confusion and need to somehow reconcile what I'm reading. Imagine for a minute you had a friend, a friend from college over the age of fifty, who was pretty heavyset. And he sent you a video of him dunking like Michael Jordan. That's sort of what this felt like.

I ring Honey and she instantly picks up, and for the next forty-five minutes she leads me through the backstory of the last four months that goes something like this:

Honey had seen a local news program about nonspeaking kids with autism learning how to communicate through something called a letterboard. She'd never heard of it, but because it was local, she figured, why not? Turns out the clinic, called Inside Voice, was about forty minutes from her house, so she starts taking Vince there a few times a week. Fast-forward a few months and, guess what. A miracle. As she puts it, "We thought 'I want juice' was his cognitive ceiling, and now he's writing all of this." This method, Spelling to Communicate (from now on referred to as "S2C"), has somehow turned Vince from a kid everyone thought had a low IQ to the guy scripting the beautiful sentences in all-caps in the screenshots. The method was invented by a woman named Elizabeth Vosseller, henceforth known as "EV," and the world headquarters for all this stuff is at her therapy practice in Herndon, Virginia.

In the autism world, every once in a blue moon, someone has a child who recovers from autism. One of my friends did Hyperbaric Oxygen therapy, and his son went on to lose his diagnosis and has already made it through college. The stories are out there, but they are rare. When you happen to have a friend who's won the "autism lottery," you are of course thrilled for them in a genuine way that perhaps only an autism parent can understand, and at the same time, you are thinking about your own child and whether this same path may be a possibility for them.

And, I'm doing this while I'm listening to Honey talk, but I am absolutely certain that Vince is some sort of freakish anomaly and Honey has somehow stumbled upon the way to unlock his extremely unique mind. I know that Jamie most certainly can't spell (because I've seen him try on a keyboard), much less string a sentence together, much less write in the complex way that Honey is telling me Vince is doing. Because I know that's not possible, I'm not going to hope for something that has no chance of happening. That'd be stupid. Honey is being annoyingly stubborn. She's giving me nothing to work with to prove my theory that Vince is an anomaly. In fact, she takes the opposite approach. "I'm going to film Vince, text it to you, and then call you back," she says. "Watch for the video."

It lands moments later. Vince is sitting there, eating dinner. I can hear Honey in the background, talking to Vince, helping him eat his dinner. He has some movement challenges, and he needs her help. His verbal responses are gibberish. He's a nonspeaker, like Jamie. He still looks like the kid I know about, the one with severe autism, the one with mannerisms. Honey calls. "See what I mean? He's still Vince, but now we know that this vibrant, beautiful mind has always been there." The whistle blows, Quinny's practice is over, I have to sign off to gather her up and get home, where a full night of homework awaits my seventh grader.

I film Jamie when I get home and send it to Honey. I guess I'm hoping for some sort of instant diagnosis. Mostly, I want Honey to put me out of my misery. For a brief second, in the 30-minute car ride home, I wondered if maybe Jamie was like Vince, but the hope felt way, way too dangerous. Honey can watch the video and tell me that, yes, of course, Jamie has the "real autism," and this can't help him. Then I can go back to this life, the one I have accepted. Enough already. She does the opposite. Her text reads:

"Jamie seems waaaay more advanced than Vince . . . seriously. I swear he is trapped in there. He's incredibly handsome, btw."

My tears start flowing. All I know for sure is we're going to Virginia. As soon as we can.

PDX

Sacred signs always come when your
soul calls out in pain or joy.

—Lawren Leo

It's Sunday, December 16th. Christmas is right around the corner. The night after my call with Honey, I was on the phone with Growing Kids Therapy Center in Northern Virginia, the place founded by Elizabeth Vosseller that started S2C. They offer out-of-towners a two-day intense visit where you have two hours of training on both Monday and Tuesday with EV. This seems like a ridiculously short amount of time for me to see or learn anything, but they've had a cancellation and we grabbed it. Who needs Christmas Break?

I'm leaning over tying Jamie's shoes, we've just made it through security at Portland International Airport (called PDX by every local), and we will soon be on the one direct flight each day that goes to Reagan National in Washington, D.C.

I hear a familiar voice. "J.B., Jamie, what's up?"

It's Lamar Hurd. If you're from Portland, you know the name: he's the voice of the Portland Trailblazers NBA basketball team. We knew Lamar before the fame, when he was a former college All-American from Oregon State coaching youth basketball. He was Sam's coach, the best coach Sam ever had, and Lamar has also organized basketball clinics at Victory, his positive attitude a great fit with all the kids.

I'm feeling extremely vulnerable about this whole idea, this whole trip. There aren't many people, outside of family, whom I would even want to see right now much less share where I'm headed, but if I had to make a list, Lamar would be at the top. He's the real deal: a real man with a huge heart, he's forever positive and giving to everyone he meets. His life force and sincerity simply radiates from him, so I consider running into him to be quite the omen.

"Where are you guys going?" he asks. Lamar is family, he's been in our lives for almost a decade, he knows Jamie, has always treated him with the utmost respect, so I spill the whole story about where we're headed. It's only been a week since I spoke with Honey, and I've been trying to learn everything I can about S2C and the prospects for Jamie.

I was fortunate to find a website called "Spellers Learn" that provides what are known as "lessons" for S2C. Basically, the teaching method of S2C is to read a lesson to a nonspeaker and then ask the nonspeaker to spell words and answer "known" questions about content from the lesson. The lesson could be "Oceans of the World" or "Abraham Lincoln," it really doesn't matter. The point is to build the connection between the child's cognition and their "motor," which means their ability to move their arm and point to the letters. Initially, the only words they are asked to spell are "known" words, which means a word that was both used and highlighted in the lesson. Over time, you slowly ask the nonspeaker increasingly challenging questions, like multiword answers from the lesson, and then finally you graduate to the big moment: seeking their opinion about the lesson.

Importantly, S2C makes a critical assumption about nonspeaking children: cognition is already there, as in fully and completely there. These kids are as smart as (probably smarter) than any "normal" kid of the same age. These lessons aren't helping the child learn how to think or process; they can already do that. The purpose they're really serving is to connect the brain to the motor, to allow these complex thoughts to come out through the letterboard by helping nonspeakers do the thing that's actually hardest: getting their body to move the way their brain wants it to. Once a child is spelling free-form the way Vince was, they are considered "open," meaning they are now open communicators who can spell fluently on the letterboard about any topic. Getting a child "open" is not only a goal of S2C, but it's also a momentous occasion for everyone involved, especially the child. The thought of this happening to Jamie is way too much for me to bear, so I simply don't consider it. I'm going to Virginia because Honey said I should. It's a giant long shot; the odds are higher that I will soon be dunking. End of thought.

After perusing the Spellers Learn website, I sent a blind email through their contact page, basically saying, "Help me, I'm new," and the woman who runs the site, Elizabeth Zielinski, responded with the kind of warmth that is all too rare:

> I would love to talk with you about our experiences with S2C. I am not a trained practitioner of the method, but I am an educational advocate who is deeply rooted in the community of trainers and practitioners. I have no financial incentives, but I am passionate because S2C has changed my own son's life. I am sure I could put you together with the right resources.

It turns out that many parents in this S2C community are like Elizabeth. They have kids with autism who have become "open" and fluent like Vince. It's radically changed their lives for the better, and they want to help other parents have the same experience. She's generous with her time on the phone, and I start to notice a pattern that starts with Elizabeth—all these parents of spellers talk about S2C very matter-of-factly, like, "Well, of course this will work for your son. He will be open in no time."

This is hard for me to understand. How do you matter-of-fact something that would represent the greatest miracle of my life, my family's life, and of course Jamie's life? But that's just what she does. She acts like Jamie's fluency is an imminent fait accompli, even though we've yet to make it to Virginia. I'm not buying it, but I'll roll with it.

Another huge theme that Elizabeth teaches me is the notion of "presuming competence" of all nonspeakers, which basically means assume every nonspeaker with autism is every bit as normal and smart as any other kid, and treat them accordingly. I aspire to do this with Jamie all the time, but I know I fall short. I don't know what he understands, and sometimes I don't make the extra effort to explain everything to him, to try and anticipate his questions, etc., because I don't know if he's tracking any of it.

But, since Elizabeth explained this "presumption of competence" idea to me, I've been making the extra effort with Jamie, and it feels good. I email her to say, "this deep dive into S2C has already changed my relationship with Jamie as I'm just giving him the benefit of the doubt that he understands everything." I can only read Elizabeth's response once because it's a hope bomb:

It's hard for me to explain how happy that makes me. You may be surprised that a stranger cares so much, and I'd understand that. But the world of autism—as you know— is just so full of injustice, misinformation, false starts, and lack of support. This is not one of those things. And as someone who knows at a visceral level what it feels like to meet your own kid, authentically, for the first time? Well, I'd have to have a heart of stone to not be moved each time a family finds this.

Mostly I'm excited for Jamie. How it must feel to be heard as he is about to be. It's life-altering, and that's not a term I use easily. I know it will work for you. I know it.

I can't wait to hear more from the other side of your visit.

I'm sharing all of this with Lamar. Presumption of competence. Getting "open." Letterboards. Spellers. All these new buzzwords of this world I never knew even existed. The fact that we may have been wrong all this time about Jamie. He's listening intently, mouth agape at times, shifting his gaze between me and Jamie, trying to take it all in. By the time I'm done with my babbling, we need to go, our flight awaits.

It's scary telling this to Lamar; he's the first person other than family who's heard about this. Do I sound like I've lost my mind? Lamar doesn't think so. "My mind is blown," he says. "Absolutely blown. I'm in this with you now, J.B., you have to keep me looped in. I'm in this with you!" He looks directly at Jamie, right into his eyes, "Good luck, Jamie, I'm rooting for you." I feel the tears well up. Lamar has always treated Jamie with respect; he instinctively presumes competence. That's hope sneaking in. I swallow hard to choke it down. I look at Jamie. He's smiling broadly.

We just make our flight.

Herndon

Everything has beauty, but not everyone sees it.

—Confucius

I hate Reston, Virginia. And I'm not just saying that, I really do hate it, which is unfortunate, because both of my parents and my only sibling, my older sister Laura, live here. In a cruel coincidence, Reston happens to border the town of Herndon, Virginia, which is where Growing Kids Therapy Center, the home of EV and S2C, is located. As I struggle to wake up at what for me is the brutally early hour of 5:00 a.m. (I'm three hours behind Eastern Standard Time in Oregon), it's already eight o'clock in the morning here, and I can hear my dad whistling and smell his extrastrong coffee brewing. It's freezing outside.

Jamie is a rock sleeping next to me in my parents' house. He sleeps like any teenager, and I'm not looking forward to waking him up. My hatred for Reston started when I was Jamie's age. Like many who live in Northern Virginia, I was a military brat; and in my case, I moved all over the world, living in six different countries. I did junior high and early high school in Tokyo, Japan, and loved every second of being there, so when my folks got moved back to the States for my junior year of high school, the reintegration was brutal, and my scars remain. I always wondered what would cause me to actually come back here—it's been decades, since my sister's wedding—and now I know: the chance for a miracle with my son.

We're still groggy as we gulp down a breakfast cooked by my always-optimistic mom, borrow my dad's car, and hit the road for Herndon. At our first light, while we're waiting to turn left, the craziest thing happens. A car careens across the median and T-bones the guy right in front of me. It's a crazy, loud, scary scene. The T-boned car jumps lanes and hits the car to the right of him, so now I'm kind of blocked in. No one seems too hurt, and there are plenty of people already on their phones calling for help, so I do a superfast four-point turn and get the heck out of there—I'm not gonna miss this appointment!

The drive is only ten minutes, and I keep thinking about the "heads-up" Elizabeth Zielinski gave me just before we departed. She wrote:

> The one thing that out of towners say they notice most about the clinic is that when you are there in the waiting area, absolutely everyone will greet your son directly. He may not answer, but it won't change the way they interact with him. No one will talk about him as if he isn't there or isn't part of the conversation. It's an incredible level of acceptance for our kids that I treasure when I am there with my son.
>
> One more thing . . . There is nothing you or your son could do or say that hasn't been done or said there before. It's the only place other than at home where I feel as though my son is completely safe and respected, even during a full-on DEFCON one meltdown. No one has to apologize for any behavior there, because everyone has shown it or watched it. That alone can take a lot of anxiety out of an experience for the students. And the parents.

If you're an autism parent, you realize how beautiful these words are. Having a place, outside of your home, where your child is truly accepted for who they are and where you can let down your hypervigilant guard for a moment is truly a rare thing. And, she's right. We roll into the Growing Kids Therapy Center (GKTC from now on), a nondescript setting of offices and learning rooms sitting just off a busy thoroughfare, and we're immediately greeted by Jeanne, the receptionist, and she doesn't give me a second look. She's entirely focused on welcoming Jamie. "Hello Jamie, it's so great to meet you, welcome, please make yourself comfortable. Elizabeth will see you very soon."

It feels great, really, to be in the background. I'm happy to play along with this charade that Jamie's fully there, although deep down I can't help but feel this is going to be another bust. It's cold. It's early. I'm exhausted from the cross-country trip and poor sleep last night. What am I doing here? Chasing a miracle? A poster on the wall catches my eye:

Once trapped inside, my thoughts are finally free.

Ugh. I can't read that again. The hope is too painful. I'm reminded of the introductory video I rewatched about S2C, starring EV, on the plane ride. She explains:

Traditionally looking at it, we had a cognitive approach first, that it was an intellectual disability in people with autism. Then it sort of switched into well there's a behavioral component to it and there's avoidance or lack of motivation or lack of caring to do well so we have to appeal at a behavioral level. But, it's not an issue of I don't understand, it's not an issue of I don't want to, it's an issue of "I can't make my body do that."

So, basically, she's throwing seventy years of autism research out the window and saying every expert in the field is wrong. They have been saying the majority of people with autism are "mentally retarded." But EV says autism isn't really about cognition. It's not something you solve behaviorally, which is what the most accepted form of autism therapy, Applied Behavior Analysis (ABA), is founded upon. These nonspeaking kids are cognitively completely intact; they just can't make their body do what they want or need it to do. The disability is a motor planning and motor execution disability. Nothing else. Like the sign in the lobby says, they are "trapped inside." It's intriguing, to say the least. She explains more about the actual teaching method:

> That's why a lot of these guys are not given credit for being as smart as they are. Spelling to Communicate helps to make a connection between intent and action. All means of communication require motor skills. Speech is really complex, it's one of the finest of the fine motors. The other complexity is the digits, and that's what we use for communication. We start by taking communication out of speech, and we teach purposeful movement by using the whole arm, taking it out of fine motor, putting it in gross motor, to be able to point to letters on an increasingly complex series of letter boards to keyboards, and that's how we give them a vehicle to express their thoughts and ideas. And, the assumption is you can and do understand me, you can and do want to learn, and we go from that position.

Simple as that, right? I realize that "matter-of-fact" vibe I've picked up on starts with her. Sure, EV, sure, let's just teach these kids how to point and, voilà, their inner genius will emerge. She does realize, right, that this would be the greatest thing that ever,

ever happened to our family, right? To discover that Jamie has a voice just like Vince would be . . . oh shit, I'm letting hope seep in again, and Jeanne interrupts my thoughts when she strides in, looks right past me, and says, "Jamie, meet Elizabeth."

Elizabeth, EV to all her friends, is immediately warm, and, as you already know, she's focused on Jamie, greeting him warmly. She seems supercalm, confident even. She greets me warmly too, and we're immediately headed back to a simple teaching room, and as the three of us walk inside I see a single desk with two chairs, a video camera on a tripod, and a chair in the back, which I presume is mine. I've already texted Lisa a picture of the "trapped inside" poster, and she texts me back with the word *Bawling*. She's hanging on my every text, and, unlike me, she's let some hope seep in, and I know it's killing her not to be here.

EV wastes no time. She sits down at the table, to Jamie's right, and begins, having already turned on the videotape. "So, my friend, this is how it's going to roll," she says. I already feel like Jamie is warm and calm. "My name is Elizabeth," she tells Jamie, and then spells it out calling out each letter in her name, "E-L-I-Z-A-B-E-T-H." She continues, "and I'm so glad you came out to see me." Then, she drops the first line that immediately causes me to weep.

"And I already know you're smart, you don't have anything to prove to me." I'm a mess, and I realize that holding back my hope has only been a superficial exercise. Has anyone ever said that to Jamie before? I sure don't think so. She keeps going. "I'm going to teach you how to do something new, totally new, that may feel a little bit weird at first." EV picks up the first "letterboard." Note that in S2C there are many types of letterboards, and Jamie is starting with the training wheels of letterboards, which are called "the three boards." Basically, each of the three boards is a hard plastic stencil board with eight letters on it, arranged alphabetically, a little bit bigger than a normal-sized piece of paper.

Just as EV picks up the stencil, Jamie smiles and lets out a belly laugh. I know this as a sign that he is feeling real joy, and I'm wishing I could understand why. EV gets Jamie to sit up straight, put both feet on the ground, picks up the first letter-board with the letters A through H on it, puts a pencil in Jamie's right hand, and says, "OK, we're going to spell my name, so poke E to start." Jamie pokes through the stenciled E without hesitation, EV guides him to pull his pencil back out, deftly switches boards to the middle board with the letters I through R on it, and then says "Poke L." Jamie does so perfectly, and they do this over and over until her entire name has been spelled. The kid is getting it, and I'm damn proud! He's smiling the whole time. After every poke of a letter, EV offers a superenthusiastic "Good!"

"OK, so here's the thing, I know, as I already said, that you are really smart and have a really great brain, but that it's hard for you to use your mouth in order to talk. It's harder for you than it is for me. I just got lucky it's really easy for me to use my mouth. But, you also have a great brain and lots of good things to say, so I'm going to teach you a different way to communicate and that's going to be to spell using your arm instead of your mouth, because it's easier to move your arm. OK?"

I'm really struggling to internalize the gravity of what she's saying, and I know this isn't the first time EV has said these words. Is this really it? Is it that simple? You're telling me these kids are all brilliant, they always have been, and they just can't get the words out? These nonspeaking kids with autism, the ones relegated to the life skills classrooms and the adult scrap heap, are all a bunch of geniuses and she's the first one to figure this out? How could this be possible? There's a nuance here, one explained to me by Elizabeth Zielinski: fine motor versus gross motor. Most communication is fine motor. Talking, writing, typing. For kids like Jamie, fine motor is very, very hard. What EV is now asking Jamie to do is gross motor. He's mostly moving his shoulder. For whatever reason, this is much easier.

EV asks him a simple question. "Jamie, I said you had a great what?" With some prompting from EV, Jamie spells the word "brain." This continues with the words "arm" and "spell," two more perfect Jamie answers to EV's simple questions.

"I like people to learn stuff while we practice this poking, so we're going to learn about the history of popcorn," EV declares. Thus begins Jamie's first experience with an S2C lesson, which is a way for Jamie to learn something while practicing the physical act of poking a pencil through the stenciled letter. As she takes Jamie though popcorn's history, she writes down and spells out loud a number of words like "popcorn" and "buttery" and "movies" and "cracker jacks." After roughly a paragraph of the lesson, she stops to ask Jamie some questions.

"What are we talking about?" Jamie pokes the word "popcorn." I'm confused. I didn't even know he could spell. At all.

"OK. And, where do we eat buttery popcorn?" EV gets Jamie to sit up straighter in his chair, get both feet flat on the floor. He pokes the word "movies." She's still having to prompt Jamie quite a bit, but it sure feels like he's tracking her and spelling the words. "And what do we eat at baseball games?" He spells "cracker jacks." Wait. What? Because of Jamie's diet, the kid has never seen a box of Cracker Jacks in his life. But he spells it without much hesitation.

"Nice, well done!" EV high-fives Jamie. This continues for more than half an hour. I notice Jamie is focused the whole time and is not having any issue remaining in his chair. Oftentimes, Jamie will need to get up and move or "stim" by shaking his arms or making loud noises when he's asked to pay attention for a long time. I'm not used to seeing him like this.

I'm also confused, because I'm sitting pretty far back, and I can't see the table. Is Jamie copying the words he sees her write? He must be. How could he possibly hear the words once in the lesson, and then spell them correctly? That doesn't make sense. Jamie doesn't have that aptitude. He's never really been taught to spell. This can't be right.

He spells "microwave," he spells "General Mills," he spells so many words I lose track, and I notice EV is really in a zone, just connected to Jamie and his poking and spelling. Positive feedback abounds. "Jamie, what year did they get the microwave popcorn patent?" Jamie spells 1981 on a number board, quick as can be. "I think you might be a numbers guy," EV smiles as she speaks, and keeps going, "I'm so proud of you, you're super-smart, and this is just the beginning, the more you practice this, the easier it will get, OK?"

EV tells Jamie she's going to talk to his dad for a moment and turns to me. I'm nervous as hell. Is she going to let me down easy? Tell me my son is a really great kid but not a candidate for this method? All I've really known is heartbreak, so there's no reason this should be any different.

"He, oh my gosh, crushed it." I'm still confused. I'm not even sure what I saw. I need EV to clarify something for me: "When you were prompting him, what was he looking at?" I'm thinking he must have been looking at the words she wrote down. She tells me he couldn't see the words, because she covers the sheet before she asks the questions. "He was giving you those answers without . . . ?" I ask. "Correct," she interrupts me, "He was spelling out of his head." I'm really struggling. "He recollected all those words from the single time you said them?" I'm still in disbelief. "Yes," EV responds. I'm in a little bit of shock.

All that comes out is, "Holy Crap." Inside, my brain is a mess. Euphoria, confusion, hope, and fear are battling it out. I look at Jamie. He's beaming.

"Jamie is a really smart guy," she says, "and our population of nonspeakers has been grossly underestimated. And, part of it is not being able to get your body to do it; it's a breakdown of the connections between the brain and the body. The brain is sending perfectly clear messages, the body is not receiving it, the body can't execute the message, that's the gist of it." I know some of this, because of the studying I've done in the past week, but seeing it for myself is something different.

EV starts sketching a brain map on a sheet of paper. I'm still processing what she's just told me about Jamie, I'm struggling to concentrate. "When you're listening to me, my sounds are going out of my mouth and into your ear and through your auditory system to this area called Wernicke's area, which is the area for comprehension. So you're understanding what I'm saying as I'm saying it, and you're interpreting those speech sounds as they come through into meaningful words," she says, explaining how you then start to form your own thoughts to respond to what you've heard.

"Broca's area is the area for expressive language, and it is your thoughts and ideas and words. So as you're listening to me, you're understanding me because of Wernecke's, but you are also having some thoughts here in Broca's, but you're not saying anything yet. Right now, these thoughts and ideas are trapped inside your head," she says, and I think I know where she's going, but it still hurts when she actually says it:

"And he has seventeen years of ideas trapped inside his head." Ugh. Can you be euphoric and in deathly pain in the same moment? I think I am. She's telling me he's always been right here.

EV continues, "The ability to communicate, which means the sharing or exchange of ideas between two or more people, requires motor—every single form of it. So with our guys, who have a primary deficit in sensory motor, which is what their biggest issue is, I don't care about the other diagnosis, the biggest issue that's affecting their life is this motor planning. All communication requires motor. So, you can use your gross motor. You could push something away that you don't want. You could kick me, you could push me away. You could punch me. Gross motor communication our guys have down pretty well. But the most robust communication requires fine motor, which is the digits or the articulators, which are all the moving parts of speech. So, in order to communicate, you have to have motor." And, as EV talks, I find myself seeing Jamie in an entirely new light, right before my eyes. He's sitting there, listening, taking everything in, and he looks extremely content, like EV is telling me something that he's known all along.

"So up here is the motor strip, which is called the primary motor cortex. Right next to it, smack right next to it, is the sensory strip. About 75 percent of the space on the motor strip is dedicated to the digits and the articulators, because they're the hardest to move. Right here, next to the motor strip, is an area called the supplemental motor cortex, and its responsible for voluntary or purposeful movement. When you have a problem with this area, it's called apraxia, and everyone we see here has some form of apraxia. For our guys with apraxia, there is a breakdown between planning and execution. What we do is we take the movement out of the fine motor of the digits and into the gross motor of the arm. And, he took to it like a champ. Speech is 100 percent motor. Language is 100 percent cognitive. They are in two different areas of the brain. So, just because the motor and speech are affected does not mean the cognition or language is affected. There's never any doubt in my mind that when someone walks into my room they can and will spell for me, that they can and do want to learn. Even seeing his engagement, oh my gosh, he's a dream to work with, he's so cooperative, so dialed in because I'm engaging both his body and his brain," and now I'm listening intently, because it's all making sense, and the years of frustration, I can actually feel them melting away, and the emotion in me, it's crawling up my throat, I'm not sure if I want to burst into tears or jump for joy, and even though I think I know the answer, I just have to ask her, I need to hear it from her.

"So, I mean, do you have any doubt that he's cognitively a seventeen-year-old?" I ask, trying to hang onto my composure.

"Zero," she responds. "Zero, like from my toenails to the top of my head, he's all here."

I don't black out, but my vision really narrows as I hear this. I'm having some sort of emotional event. It doesn't have a name, because I've never been here before. I think it might be years of suppressed hope, surging back into my body, all at once. EV says something about taking a break and seeing us again in a few hours, and before I know it we're in the car, heading to Chipotle. And everything feels different.

Dulles Airport

Miracles are not in contradiction to nature. They
are only in contradiction with what we know of
nature.

—Saint Augustine

It's Tuesday night, and Jamie and I are at Dulles Airport, waiting for our flight back to Seattle—the latest cross-country
flight I could get—before a quick twin-prop down to Portland.
It's going to be a long night: with the three-hour time change
we still won't land in Portland until after one in the morning,
but I could care less, I'm running on joyful adrenaline. It's hard
to believe that just over 48 hours ago I was in Portland Airport
talking to Lamar about our journey, and now I'm sitting here,
holding my son's hand and looking at him in a way I never have
before. As I told Lamar the story, I really didn't believe my own
words, I didn't let the possibility actually sink in, but now, now
I feel it, it's real and I know it with my heart: Jamie has always,
always been there.

After Jamie's first session, I gave Lisa a complete rundown,
or at least as much as I could, in between my tears. EV's comments about how certain she was of Jamie's cognition really
allowed my spigots to open completely, and years of unanswered
prayers and hopes all came crashing out at once. Hearing Lisa's
voice, knowing that she was in it just like I was and really the

only one who could ever understand, it was just too much, so there I sat, in a Chipotle parking lot, crying like a baby.

And, if the first session convinced EV that Jamie was cognitively all there, the second session convinced me that Jamie was, at least, much more than I gave him credit for. As Jamie settled in with EV, his belly full from our early lunch, the afternoon topic was plants, and Jamie was even more focused and independent than he had been in his first hour. He started whizzing through words, spelling "plant," chimpanzees," and, to my great surprise, "complex mechanisms." It's like you can't believe what you're seeing, and it just keeps happening, and getting better. EV asked Jamie a question, "What term means meat eating?" Jamie spelled "carnivorous." I was paying pretty close attention to the lesson, which is why her next question really caught me off guard. "Jamie, what's the opposite of a carnivore?" she asked. I'm racking my brain, nearly certain the word she was asking for had never been in the lesson. At this point, I've accepted that Jamie can spell words he's just heard and watched someone else write down, but knowing the opposite of carnivore and spelling it on his own? I wasn't prepared to believe that yet.

"Herbivore." Jamie spelled it. Just like that. "Elizabeth?" I asked meekly, "Was that word in your lesson, I don't recall hearing it?"

"No," she said, "no, it wasn't. We call that prior knowledge, I'm not surprised." And, at that point, a grown man who just turned fifty began weeping.

Today, Tuesday, EV spent more of the two sessions we had training me than working with Jamie. She explained that in order for his brain and motor to really become connected, daily practice was a must, which meant the responsibility for this really falls on the parents. I was a clumsy, clunky mess as I tried to mimic what EV was doing with Jamie, and I'd often show up with the wrong stencil board at the wrong time, to Jamie's obvious consternation. It was nerve-racking, and I was grateful EV had filmed her sessions with Jamie so I'd have something to show Lisa and to go back and remember how to do this. As our time was drawing to a close on Day 2, I was really dreading the departure from the warm, safe confines of the Growing Kids Therapy Center, and the tremendous joy it had given both of us.

For the last couple of weeks, at the behest of my newfound friend Elizabeth Zielinski, I had been trying to do a better job of talking to Jamie just like I'd talk to any other seventeen-year-old, and also to explaining to him things about the world that he might not know. Because I didn't get any feedback from Jamie, this often made me feel like I might be wasting my time, but those feelings are gone now. Sitting with Jamie now, I believe he understands me, I'm hopeful what EV believes about Jamie is true, and I have faith it's just a matter of time before Jamie is "open" fluent at using a letterboard to communicate to us about his wants, his needs, his opinions, and his feelings.

EV also taught me something that makes so much sense: never read the body language of a nonspeaking kid. The motor planning challenges that make speech impossible also mean that the body may not reflect what's going on in the mind at all. As she put it, "listening doesn't have a look." Jamie could appear preoccupied or uninterested when in fact he's listening intently. Instead, EV assures me that nonspeakers are the most acute, best listeners on the planet, because that's been their only option for so long. They are masters of absorbing information wherever and whenever they can, and they are always, always listening, so don't even worry about what you think they're thinking: you're probably wrong.

The flight to Seattle is sheer joy for me. I probably am driving Jamie nuts, but I'm talking to him the whole time about anything and everything I can think of. I'm starting to feel that we have lots of time to make up for, so why not start now? I also feel, for the first time, something other than joy. It's starting to bubble up in the background, between bouts of euphoria, and it feels like guilt. Intense guilt. How did I miss this? How did I let my son suffer in silence for so long? I slam the door on that feeling. How can I feel guilty when I just witnessed the greatest miracle of my son's life? How can I feel anything but joy? A few hours into the flight, I realize I'm exhausted. I accept it's going to be an emotional time, and I know I wouldn't trade being where I am right now for anywhere in the world. I nod off on Jamie's shoulder, desperately curious about how he is feeling right now and, for the first time ever, believing that someday soon he might be able to tell me.

Newport Beach

If you would be a real seeker after truth, it is nec-
essary that at least once in your life you doubt, as
far as possible, all things.

—René Descartes

The breakfast spread looks awesome here in Newport Beach, California. But the coffee matters more to me. It's early, and I slept like shit last night in our hotel room. It's been almost a month since we saw EV in Virginia, and Jamie and I are on the next leg of our journey down here in Southern California. Joining us today is my father, who flew in from Virginia last night to spend the next four days with us as we meet with the West Coast's leading guru of S2C, Dawnmarie Gaivin, known by all as "DM."

To be honest, I've lost some faith since the heady days spent in Herndon with EV. For the last thirty days, through Christmas break, Lisa and I have worked with Jamie every day, as instructed, going through lessons and having him spell words and answer simple "known" questions. At first, it was a lot clunkier than what Jamie was able to do with EV, but Lisa in particular has been a student of the videos of EV and seems to be perfecting her craft, and Jamie has really responded. For me, it's actually been really hard I put so much pressure on myself when I'm working with Jamie, because it feels very life or death to me, and I'm sure

Jamie can sense my intensity and anxiety. We're only clicking OK. Looking back on the thirty days, I feel we're now past where he was in Herndon, in that Jamie is smoother, faster, and more independent (requires fewer "prompts" from us) than he was.

But, and this is where the doubt has crept in, is Jamie just really good at hearing and spelling words? Perhaps this is a unique skill he's always had and he gets to display it, but that's sort of it. It's not like we're getting any insight into Jamie's inner world, intelligence, or cognition. Maybe Jamie is just the Jamie we know, with this one parlor trick that he can spell words you say to him. Herndon and EV and all her confidence about Jamie's trajectory feel very far away, and, combined with a bad night of sleep, I'm feeling a little glum.

My dad is here, and that's a good thing. He's a rock for me. I was born with a highly dependable dad, and he's never let me down. When I told him I needed him to join me for this trip, he booked his tickets that day, and now here he is. He's also a big Jamie fan, and they have always had a very loving connection. When we arrived at the hotel last night, my dad was already here, sharing a room with us, and the instant Jamie saw him he was all smiles and immediately jumped into my dad's lap, 220 pounds of love.

The S2C community is very, very small. EV has created a thorough program for certifying teachers—they all have to do things exactly the same way—and it's very structured and systematized, the goal being to ensure that every child has the time to develop the proper skills. DM was one of EV's first graduates, and her skill and talent is widely revered among the parents who know her. DM helped her own son, Evan, become fluent on the boards, and I'm thrilled to be meeting someone who is also an autism parent, because it's a bond that really no one else can understand.

We're staying in Newport Beach, because it's one of Jamie's favorite places, or at least that's what I think because we've never actually been able to ask him. We've vacationed here before, and most daylight hours are spent at the beach, with Jamie often in the ocean. We are meeting with DM for two 1-hour sessions each day for the week, so Jamie will have plenty of afternoon time to hit the beach. The 50-minute drive south to DM's offices in Oceanside goes by quickly, as I spend my time catching my dad up on the Christmas Break and everything I have learned about S2C. He probably thinks I'm crazy, but I know he'll never tell me.

The trip takes a bit longer than I thought, and we're rushing to get into DM's offices on time. Like everyone else in the S2C universe, DM greets Jamie first and focuses her positive energy on him as we file into a small therapy room, with me sitting right next to the desk with DM and Jamie, while my dad is in the back of the room. I'm hoping having my dad here was a good call and that I'm not putting too much pressure on Jamie.

DM jumps right in spelling her name, telling Jamie her nickname is "DM" and sharing the fact that she's from back East but is a happy, transplanted Californian. Jamie's spelling is really smooth and fast; I'm not sure what DM is doing differently, but Jamie looks great. He spells "bicoastal" supereasily, and DM remarks, "You're a rock star."

They immediately jump into a lesson on Ben Franklin, and Jamie smoothly spells words like "education" and "printer" and "Philadelphia." DM then decides Jamie is ready for an upgrade and switches over to what's known as the "26-letter stencil board." Basically, it's a stencil board with the entire alphabet in one place. To date, Jamie has been working with three separate boards of eight letters each, which means he could never, even if he wanted to, say something spontaneous. He's only able to respond to words that are "known" from his lesson, so his teacher can anticipate which of the three boards to present him with. The 26-letter board changes everything, because now Jamie could theoretically spell anything he wanted, which would open the door to what's known as "open communication." It's a huge step, and I'm nervous as she picks up the big board. Jamie spells "London" on the big board, without any hesitation, and DM remarks, "Great job!"

For the rest of the lesson, DM rotates back and forth between the three boards and the one giant board. Jamie seems fine with either, and I can see how focused he is. It makes me proud to see him working so hard. My dad has pretty much been cheering after each word Jamie spells right, but I'm in a different place. My inner doubts are still plaguing me, and while I'm thrilled Jamie is so smooth and accurate with his spelling, I can't help but think that he's just perfecting the parlor trick. The lesson finishes with DM asking Jamie to name a modern superstition. He spells, "Walking under a ladder." Yes, she said it during the lesson, but that's the first time I've seen him spell a sentence, which is pretty cool.

After an hour break, we're back at it. For this hour, DM is really just training me, so I'm getting exhausted. My nerves about working with Jamie are coming up, and it's clear that he is nowhere near as fast spelling with me as he is with DM. The S2C people call the interaction a "dance," and I'm the crappy dance partner. It's humbling. To his credit, Jamie is a great sport, and we make it through the hour. We're no closer to "open" communication, but I can't wait to hit the beach.

Day two starts a lot like day one. Jamie is spelling smoothly, and he and DM are working their way through a lesson on "Shuffleboard." He spells words like "billiards" and "tournament" without hesitation, and I'm watching intently. DM is using the 26-letter stencil more than she was yesterday, and Jamie is definitely getting better. In fact, he's faster on the big board, and he seems to really want to impress DM. Out of the blue, she asks Jamie a math question: "If red scores 9 and blue scores 5, what's the net score?" DM puts a number stencil board in front of Jamie, and he instantly pokes "4." What? I'm stunned. I didn't know he could do math! She tries another, "If red scores 5 and blue scores 12, what's the net score?" Jamie immediately pokes 7. My dad and I look at each other across the room. We both look puzzled. What's going on?

DM grabs the big board again, turns to Jamie, and asks, "What should your shuffleboard name be?" I'm confused. This obviously isn't a question from the lesson. She sees my face and quickly says, "This is a low-risk open." What she means is this is indeed an "open" question—a question that requires open communication because there is no set answer—but it's one where the stakes are pretty low, at least according to her. You see, DM has the same vibe all the other S2C people have, that matter-of-fact "of course your son will have a miracle" vibe, so for her, this is nothing more than a "low-risk open." I, however, am seeing the gravity of this question, and I sense my dad is too, and we're both leaning in for his response. It feels more like my entire existence is at stake.

Jamie pokes J, then A, and I realize he's going to spell his name. He's known how to spell his name for a long time, so this is nothing new. She said spell a shuffleboard name, he heard name, he's spelling his name. Big deal. He finishes the "E" in Jamie, and I figure he's done and sit back in my chair. Oh well, all good. But he's not done.

DM calls out the next letters as he spells them, "N-O-T-O-R-I-O-U-S, Notorious, L Y, Notoriously, S-T-R-O-N-G, Strong." I can't believe it. My dad lets out a long "Holy moly, dude." DM makes sure she heard him right: "Is your shuffle-board name Jamie Notoriously Strong?" Jamie spells, "Yes." I'm staring at my beautiful son. But, things feel different. I'm seeing him as I've never seen him before. Jesus, I don't think I have any idea how deep this kid really is. Notoriously Strong? I'm dumb-founded. It's a great feeling, though. The doubt is dissipating. Quickly!

We take a much-needed (for me) two-hour break. I'm on the phone with Lisa to give her the minute-by-minute account. I hold off giving her the punchline until the very end of our call. I can barely get the words out: "He named himself Jamie Notoriously Strong." She's done; all I can hear is her crying.

Our afternoon session involves a beautiful story about the disabilities activist Haben Girma, and Jamie seems super-engaged. He's getting even better on the 26-letter board. The lesson ends with DM explaining how Haben hopes to start a revolution for people with disabilities. DM looks at me and then asks Jamie a question, "What would you name her revolution?" I look at my dad. Here we go again. Open communication time. Jamie pokes out:

"Inclusion all around the world."

I do a double take. He just wrote "Inclusion all around the world." I watched him write it, I saw him poke every letter. DM holds the board perfectly still. It's him doing the writing. It's so wonderfully incisive, such powerful self-advocacy. From my son, the nonspeaker whom everyone has discounted, including me. What level of intellect is required to create that beautiful name for a revolution? How much thought has Jamie put into topics like this? Has this emerging brilliance I'm seeing always been there, processing the world so artfully, even if no one else ever knew?

Things are feeling good, really good. Day two has been the best day ever with Jamie. His shuffleboard name has sent me and Lisa to the moon and back. The beach is sunny and crisp, he splashes in the water, and I stand with my dad. He's blown away, too, and starting to believe just like I am. Maybe Jamie is just like Vince.

Day three begins, and I'm already pumping with adrenaline, the anticipation of what extraordinary things will be unveiled about my son today. Doubt has taken a serious back seat, and I'm overwhelmed with the joy of learning who Jamie really is. Today's first lesson is "Coat of Arms," and Jamie is getting even faster at spelling. DM asks Jamie to think about designing his own family coat of arms. "Give me an adjective to describe your family?" Jamie spells, "Resilient." DM explains that among animals, the bull most closely represents resiliency. She explains, "The animal usually holds an object representing an ideal the family stands for. What's yours?" Jamie spells, "Truth." What the hell? What is going on here? It feels like each new question simply expands the possibility for this kid's brilliance, his eloquence, his heart! How is this happening?

We have a longer break today and find our way to downtown Carlsbad and hang out at a very hip outdoor juice bar. It's January, but it's simply beautiful out, and I'm feeling great, thrilled my dad is here, seeing Jamie emerge. My dad, he's every bit as stunned as I am. He's looking at Jamie, just like I am, more smitten than ever with his amazing grandson. Neither of us really has the words to explain what's going on in this moment. Maybe this is what lottery winners feel like: I don't really know.

The afternoon lesson is a rougher pill to swallow. It's all about the Boston Red Sox team of 2004 that finally won a World Series. It turns out DM is an insufferable Red Sox fan, which will be hard for me and my dad, both Yankee fans—and I'm pretty diehard. Jamie is flowing on the big board, and the open questions are coming easily. DM asks, "What's another word for a fierce sports rivalry?"

"Intense competition," Jamie spells.

"Let's use the word *scrappy* in a sentence," DM requests.

"My mom is the scrappiest woman on Earth," Jamie spells. He turns and looks at me. I give him a huge smile, I really have no words. I text to Lisa, "You better sit down for this one." My own tears are flowing freely. I don't dare look at my dad; I'm sure he's a mess.

I realize I don't really know if Jamie knows I'm a Yankee fan. Yes, it's becoming very clear that there is a hell of a lot more going on in him than we ever knew, that Jamie is very, very capable of independent thought and stringing words together. Certainly before we saw EV and even before this trip to DM, if you'd asked me if Jamie knew I was a Yankee fan, I'd say, "no." That's too many abstract thoughts that would have to be put together. Does he even know what pro sports means? I watch SportsCenter every night and yes, he's often sitting with me, but does he track any of that? No, I wouldn't have thought so.

The lesson is coming to a close. It's been an amazing day. Lisa texts me that she had to pull over after the "scrappy" note hit her text, that she was crying too hard to drive. With a minute left in the lesson, DM turns to Jamie and asks, "What are your thoughts on all of this? The lesson I mean?"

Jamie spells, "The Sox won, but the Yankees are champs in my family." The room is silent. The implications of what he just said are only slowly sinking in. I make eye contact with my dad. Big mistake: two grown men are now blubbering like babies.

Palm Springs

The president needs to realize nonspeakers think,
feel, and learn just like everyone else.

—Jamie Handley

Our final day with DM exceeded all expectations. I'm back in the car now with Jamie, late on Friday afternoon. The good-bye with my dad was both tearful and joyful. How are you supposed to feel after witnessing a miracle? I think he's still trying to figure it out, and the flight home to Virginia will no doubt be a joyful one. I'm comforted by that. My dad is eighty this year, and I know that the unsettled and murky future with Jamie causes him a lot of stress. He worries about me. I know he's worrying less right now.

I'll start with the punchline about today, the thing Jamie said in the final minutes of his final session that, for me, pretty much removed whatever shred of doubt I had that Jamie was everything Honey, EV, Elizabeth Zielinski, and DM have been telling me he is. I loved it so much that it's the quote opening this chapter, so read it again for yourself. It was in Jamie's response to this question from DM: "If writing a letter to the president explaining autistics are misunderstood, what would you say?" As Jamie wrote these words, I found myself swelling with pride, hope, joy, happiness, and optimism all at once. My beautiful son wasn't just fully there, he is becoming an advocate for others like him, too. He's eloquent, compassionate, incisive, funny, and wise. Words defy how good it felt. Perhaps Lisa put it best, in a reply text to me after I shared what he had spelled in the lesson. She said, "I feel like the darkness has lifted."

Earlier in the same session, somewhat out of the blue, Jamie had an emotional outburst and bit his arm. This is something we see with Jamie during times of anxiety or frustration. I'd say, perhaps 20 percent of the time we have a pretty good idea of why Jamie is frustrated, but the other 80 percent we are only left guessing and soothing him, hoping the mood passes soon. It's incredibly frustrating to not know why Jamie is having a hard time. And, for the first time in seventeen years, DM is sitting right there to ask him what's going on, so she does. "What are you feeling right now, Jamie?" she asks.

"Worried about leaving here and returning to three boards only," he spells. And, who wouldn't be? The poor kid, he finally has the chance to share his own thoughts and feelings, but when he leaves here, guess what. It's back to his old life because DM is literally the only person on the planet right now who's gotten these words out of Jamie. What if no one else can? DM allays these fears, explaining the process of getting "open" with others, including me and Lisa. I remind Jamie that we will be coming down to see DM every two weeks for the foreseeable future. Jamie responds, "Sure, that's great." He seems better.

The road is windy and beautiful between Oceanside, where we started this trip, and Palm Springs, where we're headed. It's one of my favorite weekends of the year, the Sandstorm lacrosse tournament in Palm Springs, and Jamie and I are going to meet Lisa and Quinny at the home we've rented near the fields. Sam played in this tournament for years, and now it's Quinny's turn. It's January, the sun is shining, and I feel the adrenaline and joy just pulsating through my body. At times like this, music is my favorite drug, and luckily Jamie shares these genes. He also seems to have developed my passion for old school hip-hop, although I haven't asked him that yet, so I am absolutely cranking the tunes as we drive. "Changes" by Tupac comes on, perhaps Jamie's favorite song, and we are at full decibel. Jamie is an enthusiastic dancer, and it brings me great joy to see him grooving hard and sharing in the moment.

I think back to our final lesson, before Jamie crafted his incredible note to the president. DM resumed a discussion of Jamie's family coat of arms and asked him a question, "What would be your family motto?" I was hanging onto Jamie's every poke, every one of these great questions seeming to bring a new profound insight.

"World-changing optimists," he spelled, with a confident grin. Unbelievable. In our first session this morning, I witnessed Jamie demonstrate a level of thoughtfulness and clarity that surprised me, despite my growing expectations for what Jamie was capable of. The study lesson was "Slam Poetry," and DM walked Jamie through its origins, the competitions, how it's structured, etc. At one point, she put on a short video of an actual poetry slam by Marshall Davis titled "Touchscreen." It's a powerful critique of how much our phones have disconnected us from life and one another. It's also sophisticated and delivered with a staccato rhythm that forced me to concentrate—some of the references are pretty nuanced. Jamie didn't appear to really be watching it, so I wondered if he was internalizing anything. Remember when I warned against trying to read body language? I forgot to take that advice. "What did you think of the Touchscreen poem?" DM asked.

"Not too shabby," Jamie responded. DM replied, "Anything else you want to say?"

Jamie spelled, "Lost human touch in a digital world is sad."
Mind blown.

It's been over two hours on the road, and we've descended
into the valley of Palm Springs. It's dark now. My euphoria hasn't
subsided. I can't begin to really express how much joy and hope
I am feeling. I'm also in awe of Jamie. He's so wise. He's funny.
I'm also starting to see something else: he's extremely generous.
After he wrote the note to the president, the session was winding
down, and DM asked if he had any final thoughts or questions.
Yes, he told DM, he did, "Thank you, Dawnmarie," he spelled,
and then he gave her a big hug. She asked him if he'd pose for
a picture. He spelled, "Yes." She explained that she'd like him
to hold up a small greaseboard with his word for 2020 written on it, would that be OK? Jamie sat back down and spelled
"Opportunities."

Lisa is leaning against her rental car in the driveway of our
rented home, waiting for us. I can't even imagine how excruciating it's been for her to have to live this whole week remotely, this
week when our son was returned to us. As my headlights hit her,
I can see that she's already sobbing. The reunion is intense, I'm
sobbing too, the shared grief escaping both of us. Neither of us
will let go of Jamie, and he's tucked his head in tight to us both,
snuggling while standing.

Elizabeth Zielinski had warned me back in December that
the process of becoming "open" can be very emotional for the
kids. Kind of understandable, right? In Jamie's case, more than
seventeen years of being misunderstood and not being able to
tell people how you're really feeling or show them how smart you
are. How would *you* feel? It's not even a fair question, because
how can someone who's been able to speak even relate? I know
I can't.

Jamie and I are exhausted, and I think he will nod off pretty quick. I'm lying in bed with him when suddenly I realize he's starting to whimper. Pretty soon, the whimpers turn to wails, and before I know it, Jamie is crying harder and louder than I've ever seen him. Lisa rushes in, followed by Quinny, and we're all on the bed, draping ourselves all over Jamie to try and give him comfort. The tears flow. Yes, I'm frustrated, I wish DM were here so she could ask him exactly why he's crying. But I think I know. Elizabeth prepared me. Yes, it hurts to hear him wail, but it also affirms for me that this is it, it's really happening. Jamie is Vince, and he always was, and here he comes.

The Pearl District

Quiet people have the loudest minds.
—Stephen Hawking

It's been two weeks since our miraculous trip to see DM. It's early and there's a chilly bite in the air. I'm walking through Portland's hip and trendy Pearl District, on my way to my office. Well, sort of on my way. Honestly, I've been walking now for nearly an hour, mostly in circles, trying to calm my mind. It's Tuesday morning, and Lisa is down in Newport with Jamie. It's her turn, her first chance to take Jamie to see DM, and so far every text I get from her is a new, revelatory miracle that tells us something else about the incredible depth and wisdom of Jamie's amazing mind and soul.

Hearing Lisa's text chime has become my favorite drug, and it's hard for me to concentrate as I eagerly await the next high. This week, I have to get up extra early to take Quinny to school, which is normally Lisa's job. The "divide-and-conquer" approach to raising our kids has forced each of us to specialize in the routines of one of our kids, and I've always had Jamie and Lisa has always had Quinny. This means I know very little about helping Quinny get ready for school. It sounds weird when I ask Quinny, "What do you usually have for breakfast?" But here we are. Lisa and I joke that we've raised three only children, because our kids have in many ways each grown up in their own world.

As I drove Quinny to school today, I realized this miraculous time for our family is both confusing and a little isolating for her. Even more than her older brother, Sam, Quinny has borne the brunt of the autism life. All she's known is a world where her parents are stressed and worried about her older brother. The relationship between Jamie and Quinny is hard to describe, because the lack of communication has led to the two of them basically living in different silos, despite sharing the same house. Quinny has found a way to soldier on during the many times her parents have been distracted or consumed by Jamie's challenges. She's incredibly organized and independent and always on top of her schedule, what needs to be packed, etc., in case her parents get lost in a stress-induced haze. Now, out of the blue, her brother has become a miraculous celebrity among our extended family, and I know she's struggling between being thrilled for Jamie but being once again the forgotten child. I explain to her that I see this clearly, that having mixed feelings is very normal, and that I love her. She's thirteen, so what I get in return is a quick "I'm fine." She leaves my car and is quickly enveloped by a gaggle of excited friends. It's far from perfect, but I take some comfort knowing that it's only getting better from here.

Yesterday, DM welcomed Lisa to her office for the first time and started Jamie off with a lesson about the relationship between the gastrointestinal system and autism. Jamie easily spelled words like "peristalsis," "hydrochloric acid," and "esophagus." She asked him what he thought it means when someone is described as anal-retentive. Jamie responded, "It might mean that they can't let much go." That made me laugh. The afternoon lesson was about Louis Braille and his invention of Braille for the blind. DM asked Jamie if he thought he could learn Braille. "Not really, I don't hardly have the patience." She asked Jamie which personal qualities Louis Braille might have had that allowed him to invent something so important.

His response? "He was never entering his disability feeling sorry for himself."

It's hard to express how words like that, written by my own son, make me feel. It's clear that Jamie has processed many intense feelings and somehow, in the midst of the entire world misunderstanding him, found his own philosophy toward life. He hasn't let his disability break his spirit, and I'm awed, amazed, humbled, heartbroken, and just plain in love with this amazing kid all at once.

In DM's afternoon lesson on the topic of resiliency, she walked Jamie through the life of Canadian neuroscientist Brenda Milner and her research about the personal qualities that make some people more resilient than others. DM asked Jamie what Dr. Milner credited for her own long and happy life. Jamie responded, "Stimulation of her mind."

DM then asked Jamie, "What would you develop or change in the world?" Lisa prefaces Jamie's response to DM with this text: "Heartbreaking!" Then she sends me his reply:

"I'd make nonspeakers have the opportunity to meet you and get free from their prisons of silence."

Ouch. Prisons of silence? Good God. He's seventeen. That really stings—my heart bleeds for Jamie. Simultaneously, thank you, universe; thank you, God; thank you, everyone that Jamie can now tell us this. It hurts, wow, it really hurts. The alternative is even worse, however. At least we're talking about this "prison of silence" in the past tense.

This morning, Lisa's younger sister, Kricken, arrived from Portland to attend the sessions with DM, bear witness, and keep Lisa company. Having my dad in the room a few weeks ago was definitely helpful for me, if only to affirm for me that the miracle

I was witnessing was real. DM's first lesson covers the story of William Lishman, a.k.a. "Father Goose," a dynamic naturalist, sculptor, filmmaker, and humanitarian who suffered from dyslexia. I'm starting to see a wonderful, empowering theme to all these lessons, and Jamie is certainly responding. At the end of the lesson, DM asks Jamie what he would title his own autobiography.

"Earnestly underestimated."

I immediately hear from my sister-in-law, Kricken, via text: "Your son blows my mind. He's a brilliant buddha."

In the afternoon, DM walks Jamie through a lesson about Rosa Parks. She asks Jamie why he thinks the bus boycott was so effective. Jamie spells, "There is strong influence when the money stores dry up." DM shifts the lesson to ask Jamie a more personal question, "Name a commonly held belief around autism that you would like to change."

I'm sitting at my desk as these words hit my phone, Lisa is texting me real time so it almost feels like I'm there. I see DM's question and think to myself, "This should be good!" And, Jamie doesn't disappoint:

"Right now I enjoy the prospect of helping others see how smart nonspeakers really are."

It's Friday morning now, the week has become a blur of tears, heartache, and fascination, every text from Lisa another hit of euphoria and insight helping me better grasp the remarkable depths of Jamie's mind. My nights have been spent on the phone with Lisa, rehashing every second of the lessons, with Kricken chiming in from the background about how deeply moved she has been watching her nephew in action.

These lessons are helping me better appreciate the motor deficiency and the huge role it plays in the disability of autism for nonspeakers. EV explained this concept back in December, this idea that there is a "brain-body disconnect" and that non-speakers simply cannot get their body to do what their mind wants. "The motor" is a commonly used term with all the S2C practitioners, and I'm starting to understand why. Here's a simple example: Jamie has something known as "apraxia," which basically means it's hard for him to get words out of his mouth. That's motor planning, not cognition. He knows what he'd like to say, he always has, he just can't say it. Through DM, we also learn that Jamie also has "ocular apraxia" which means it's very hard for Jamie to get his eyes to go where he wants them to go. How can she tell? Well, first, it's extremely common with all the nonspeakers she teaches, but she's also able to watch Jamie's eyes struggle as they bounce all over the letterboard to find letters, and she has the benefit of learning from her own son Evan, who's been a fluent speller for years and struggles with the same issue.

"We take it for granted that our eyes go where we want them to," she explains, "but with nonspeakers that's rarely the case. It's very hard for them to get their body to do what they want it to do. There is static between the brain and the motor, and that's the real disability. It impacts the eyes, so people think our kids can't read, but what's actually true is they can't get their eyes to do what they want them to."

On Thursday, DM took Jamie through a lesson specifically about motor differences and the nonspeaking writer Ido Kedar, author of a book called *Ido in Autismland*. She shared Ido's perspective on what are known as "stims" (repetitive behaviors) and how Ido uses his stims to help keep his body and mind regulated. She asks Jamie, "Can you think of a way stimming may help a person's sensory system?" Jamie spells, "It reaches the insatiable inner movement-seeking beast." She asks Jamie if he has any compulsions that he'd like help with. "I can't stop how I stress out because then I bite my arm compulsively" is his response. "Are you open to the idea of your parents helping you with that?" DM asks Jamie. "Yes, need their help," he responds. So many mysteries about Jamie and his inner life are being resolved. Stimming. Arm biting. We never knew for sure what was going on in Jamie's head. It's being spelled out for us, little by little, by Jamie himself. It's surreal. Life is a gift right now, a giant gift.

DM also took Jamie though a lesson about Stephen Hawking. He provokes an important question. We all accept that Stephen Hawking was brilliant, despite his inability to get his body to do what he wanted, due to his ALS, right? Is believing the same thing is happening with nonspeakers really that big a leap? DM asks Jamie how Stephen Hawking might have felt when diagnosed with ALS at twenty-one. "Horrible," he answers. "How do you think he felt fifty years later about his life?" she asks. Jamie spells, "Satisfied."

DM asks Jamie what a legacy is. Jamie spells, "What your memory of accomplishments will be after you die." DM asks Jamie what he would like his legacy to be.

"I have time to decide. Right now I'm going to learn spelling to communicate and suck up all the knowledge I can." So much wisdom!

It's finally Friday afternoon, and DM is taking Jamie through a variety of open questions, no longer using a lesson to guide her. I'm back in the Pearl District and on my way to Peet's to grab a coffee when Lisa's text hits my phone: "Sit down for this one." When I texted the same thing to Lisa two weeks ago, it was a doozy, and I feel a rush of energy through my body at the anticipation. I find the closest bench on the corner right in front of Whole Foods, take a deep breath, and stare intently at my phone awaiting the next text. It arrives: "Q: we've studied a number of people this week who overcame their disabilities to accomplish great things. Can you relate?" As Lisa later explained, Jamie got really focused after hearing this question, the speed of his spelling increased, and as it became clear what Jamie was spelling, Lisa found herself simply inconsolable. Here's how Jamie responded:

"I don't like to hate autism, however, it has had a toll on my mom and dad. Having family who will move mountains to help me makes me the luckiest human being born."

Oh wow. This kid, just look at him, the grace, the love, the perspective—and we almost never knew this?! My heart just shattered into a million pieces and swelled up to 100 times its size simultaneously. Lisa texts me, "He's just so amazing. Bawling." Jamie's Aunt Kricken sends me a text, too: "Your son is making me cry like a baby. Mascara everywhere."

College Park

My man, Sammy. You never cease to bring you're
A-game. I'm sure this weekend won't be much dif-
ferent. Thanks for taking me onto the field in spirit
on your lightning fast feet. I'm so proud to be your
sibling. Now go make history. Love, Jamie.

—Jamie Handley

It's February 14th, Valentine's Day, and Jamie and I are settling into our hotel after a cross-country flight from Los Angeles. Life has been a whirlwind since our first trip to see DM. Lisa and I have now made plans to alternate weeks where each of us takes Jamie down to see her, and Jamie and I just finished squeezing in our two days. We will spend the weekend on the East Coast and head back down to SoCal late Sunday for three more days with DM next week.

Right now, Lisa and I have another priority, which is being present at Sam's lacrosse games. Sam's freshman season, last Spring, was a surreal whirlwind of cross-country trips for Lisa and me as we tried to have at least one of us present for all of his games. As an Oregon boy, Sam is a bit of an anomaly in lacrosse, which remains an Eastern game. He surprised every-one, including us and probably himself, by being national fresh-man of the year, Ivy League Rookie of the Year, and a first-team All-American. This year, Sam will have a target on his back. He

broke all of Penn's rookie scoring records, and he opens tomorrow against the vaunted University of Maryland, a perennial
powerhouse in lacrosse.

Jamie hasn't been to many of Sam's games—last year he
made two—but times are changing. Sam has been stuck at college for this communication miracle. I really wanted him to
witness Jamie spelling for himself, so we've decided to make
the arduous journey without losing any momentum with DM.
Unfortunately, DM remains the only person on the planet Jamie
is "open" with, so we're always eager to get back down to SoCal
as quickly as we can. Hearing Jamie speak has become our favorite drug.

Today, before we raced north and got on a plane to
Maryland, we actually squeezed in two lessons with DM. During
the final lesson, I asked DM if she would ask Jamie to write a note
to Sam. You can see Jamie's handiwork at the beginning of this
chapter, the first communication Sam has ever received from his
little brother. For years, Sammy has played lacrosse with Jamie's
initials—JHH—written on his cleats, and I was thrilled to see
Jamie make reference to that fact, just one of the many small
details of life it's becoming clear Jamie has always noticed.

When we arrived this morning, DM had a special surprise
for us. Her son Evan, a fluent speller, was there to greet us, and
she'd written a brand-new lesson titled "East Coast West Coast
Rap Rivalry." Evan, just a year younger than Jamie, was also a
big old-school hip-hop fan, so the lesson resonated with both
of them. For Jamie, this was the first time he'd ever met another
speller, and I could tell he was nervous. I sat enraptured as two
beautiful, intelligent, remarkable boys talked to each other
like normal teenage "dudes." It's noteworthy that Evan really
struggles to stay still for long periods of time. He needs to move
his body frequently in order to be able to spell, so he generally

takes many more breaks than Jamie while spelling. I found this encouraging for the parents who might be looking at their non-speaker right now and saying, "that's great for Jamie, but it will never work for us." DM tells me this is common. Most parents of nonspeakers underestimate their kids, something I was certainly guilty of. I didn't even think Jamie could spell! DM tells me that's what most parents think.

The lesson began, and DM walked Evan and Jamie through the growing feud between rival record labels on each coast. She played the boys some of the lyrics from Tupac's song "Hit 'Em Up," a lyrical diatribe against the East's Bad Boy Records. DM asked the boys what they thought of the lyrics. Evan responded first, "Ballsy. Little room for misunderstanding." Jamie chimed in to support Evan, "That's true, Evan. It returned the volley to Bad Boy."

And this is how it went, two boys with so much in common, discussing a shared love and supporting each other. DM asks Jamie what part of Tupac's lyrics would have been the most offensive to Puff Daddy and Biggie? Jamie answers, "Lyrics about your wife or your mama really sting." Evan chimes in, "Total truth." It was beautiful to watch. Evan's final words to Jamie? "I have mad respect for you." The beauty of these beautiful teenage boys, both cast aside and painfully misunderstood by mainstream society, it was almost too much to bear. I feel awestruck to be in their presence.

In our final session, a lesson about "Unrequited Love" in honor of Valentine's Day, Jamie raised his game, once again. Out of the blue, Jamie spells out the following thought:

"All of this spelling today has given me a real longing for friends like Evan. Maybe next time last longer? How about if you come to Portland soon?" Instant tears for me. My beautiful boy, deprived for so long, just wants what we all want: friendship and camaraderie. He wants DM to pack it up and cart Evan up to live beside us.

I guess DM hadn't seen me cry enough today, because she raises the stakes, by asking Jamie to do a Valentine fill-in-the-blanks: "I know____loves me because____." She asks him to go through his whole family, one by one, and he does.

I know my mom loves me because she never lost hope that somehow I would speak.

I know Sammy loves me because he is my most loyal fan.

I know Quinny loves me because she virtually lives in the world of autism and never complains.

I quickly texted each of these to Lisa. It was hard to type through the tears. I wasn't sure I could take one about me.

I know my dad loves me because he is my ride or die homie.

Slayed! And, for those of you who need a lesson in hip-hop slang, being someone's "ride or die homie" is perhaps the greatest compliment I could be paid. As the Urban Dictionary explains, "Ride or Die" means "when you are willing to do anything for someone you love or someone you really appreciate in your life."

Remember that emerging generosity in Jamie that I mentioned? Well, he did it again. DM was finishing the lesson when Jamie motioned for her to bring the board back to him. He clearly had something else to spell, and he poked out:

I know Dawnmarie loves me because you make time to write rap lessons for me and E to enjoy.

This kid! It's crazy, really. We are taught, very incorrectly I now believe, that kids with autism miss social cues, that they aren't savvy with interpersonal dynamics, and yet, I'm watching Jamie demonstrate extraordinary sensitivity and awareness of those around him. Between him and Evan, they destroy so many of the stereotypes and oft-repeated "facts" about nonspeakers. These guys aren't cognitively disabled. They are extremely smart. They aren't socially clueless. They are sensitive and generous. Why haven't we known this?

It's Saturday morning now. Jamie and I are seriously sleep deprived. We meet my mom, dad, sister, and my sister's son and daughter and head to the stadium at the University of Maryland. It's freezing, and we're all bundled up. Mercifully, we find seats inside the stadium with heat lamps overhead and settle in for the game. I'm always nervous to watch Sam play, but things are very different now. The stress of Jamie has been replaced with joy, and I realize how happy I am to be surrounded by family settling in to watch my oldest son pursue his passion. It's also amazing to sit next to Jamie knowing full well he knows exactly what's going on. Sam was walking through campus yesterday when he got the text from me with a picture of Jamie's note, and he said he had to sit down on the spot to muffle the crying and regain his composure.

Maryland is ranked #3 in the country and Penn is #8, so the game is being televised, and the stakes feel high. As a sophomore, Sam is now expected to carry the offensive load for Penn, and he doesn't disappoint, scoring the first goal of the game. By the end of the third quarter, we're up, 15–11, and it feels like our game to lose. Somehow, we do just that, as Maryland outscores us, 6–0, in the final quarter to win, 17–15. Sam has a great game, scoring three goals and adding two assists, but, oddly, Sam sits on the bench during the game's crucial final two minutes, and he appears to be in quite a bit of pain.

I'm waiting for Sam at the postgame team tailgate, and I'm nervous to find out what's wrong. He comes out of the lockers, and he's not looking too happy. "It's just my ribs, Dad, I'm sure I'll be fine." I know how painful ribs can be, so it makes sense. I confirm that the trainer gave him a thorough look. Sam reassures me he'll be fine, and we hug very gently. He doesn't think he broke them, but he looks incredibly uncomfortable and really pale. He heads for the team bus back to Philadelphia, and Jamie and I give our farewells to my family and jump in our rental car. While I was excited for the game, I'm more excited for Sam to get the chance to see his brother in action, so we will see each other tonight in Philly for dinner and then some time in our hotel room, where Jamie can show Sam how he spells. No, he won't be able to spell openly the way he can with DM, but I just want Sam to see it and relive all the amazing words we have from our time with DM. It's going to be awesome.

Penn Presbyterian

You never know how strong you are until being strong is your only choice.

—Bob Marley

Jamie and I are checked in at the Inn at Penn right across the street from the University of Pennsylvania. Sam has called me twice from the team bus on the way home from Maryland complaining of intense pain. His coach and trainer have loaded him up with aspirin, but he still feels awful. We're about half an hour ahead of him, so I tell him let's grab dinner right away. I offer to bring Jamie and just go to his apartment, but he insists he can make it to the restaurant, which is only a few blocks away for him. It's already 8 p.m., and we agree to meet at the Tap House at 8:30 p.m.

Sam looks terrible when he makes it to our table. Something isn't right. "The last time I ate was before the game," he tells me. The game was at 1p.m. Sam eats like a horse, he's 6'5", 230 pounds. OK, maybe he's just deathly hungry. We order him a pizza, and he snarfs the whole thing. "Feel better?" I ask. "Maybe, I don't know," Sam responds. He's distracted, distant. "I've got to go to the bathroom." Sam heads off.

After a couple minutes have passed, my parent alarm goes off, and Jamie and I head for the bathroom. Sam has puked his pizza, he seems a little delirious, sitting next to the toilet. "I need to go to the hospital," he tells me. We beeline out of there, I call for an Uber as we walk, and we head for the closest ER at the Hospital of the University of Pennsylvania, which is only four minutes away. The ER is packed—it's Friday night. The intake coordinator takes Sam around the corner to grab some vitals. Sammy is back soon. "I'm next up," he says. Huh? This place is so crowded, what's going on? My theory is he's insanely dehydrated and probably has a cracked rib.

The call for Sam is nearly instant, and as the sliding doors to the ER open, there are six doctors standing there, and they all seem very serious. Jamie is locked into my arm, and I reflexively tell him, without believing a word of it, "It's going to be fine."

Sam's immediately put on an IV, and they are running a sonogram on him. One of the docs is serving as interpreter for me and trying to keep me calm. "His blood pressure was very low. The most likely explanation is that he injured his spleen." I know the spleen is an organ, and that's about where my knowledge ends, but I vaguely remember that athletes who rupture their spleens need to get to the ER quickly. Sammy was injured almost eight hours ago.

Each time the doctor tells me something, I turn and explain it to Jamie and try to reassure him that things are fine, which is getting harder to say as the number of doctors increases. The nice doc informs me they want to move Sam to Penn Presbyterian, which is only six blocks away, because they have an elite trauma unit standing by for emergency surgery. I'm in robot-dad mode at this point; whatever panic I should be feeling has been suppressed. If you've been through something with your child, you get it—there will be time to deal with the emotions later. Not now. "Mr. Handley, there's some traffic, we think we are going to helicopter Sam over there." Jesus Christ, I now realize how serious this is, and at the last minute they decide to take the ambulance, so Sam, Jamie, and I pile in, and we're off, sirens blazing.

The ambulance tech explains that when we hit Penn Presbyterian, they are racing Sam straight into surgery, no time to check in, so say your good-bye right now. Throughout this whole thing, Sam has been calm and strong, and that doesn't change now. We lock hands, tell each other, "I love you," and the doors explode open to another group of docs waiting for Sam, and he's swallowed by the building before Jamie and I can even get out of the ambulance. All we can do now is wait.

I finally know Jamie can understand everything, and here we are in the most stressful moment of either of our lives. It's actually a source of comfort that I can tell Jamie exactly what's going on, knowing he can understand everything. Sam's getting a splenectomy, which means his entire spleen will be removed. It's very dangerous to injure your spleen, because it's often missed, like Sam's was, and you can bleed to death. But the surgery has an extremely high recovery rate. Young and incredibly fit, Sam will be fine. Jamie seems stressed, and I don't want him to have to sit here and suffer. My dad and sister are in a car right now barreling toward Philly from Virginia. They jumped into their car to be with us as soon as I let them know we were heading to the ER. I call several of Sam's teammates, and within minutes eight of his teammates arrive, which brings me to tears. Two of Sam's teammates—Piper Bond and B.J. Farrare—know Jamie pretty well from a visit to Oregon last summer, so they agree to take him back to the hotel, settle him down, and put him to bed, knowing that my dad and sister will relieve them soon.

I'm told surgery may take up to four hours, and I'm on the phone with Lisa telling her everything. She and Quinny are in Portland and already booked on the first flight out in the morning when Dr. Brian Smith busts open the door on the opposite side of the empty waiting room and yells to me, "He did great, he's fine!" Lisa can hear it on the phone, and now we're both crying. I hear Lisa tell Quinny the news, and she starts wailing, crying with relief.

Dr. Smith and a very kind nun walk me back to see Sam. Minutes later, I'm hovering over my baby boy, in a giant postop room with just one nurse, a bunch of wires and tubes hooked up to Sam, and a new 12-inch scar the length of his abdomen. He's too drugged up to say much, and I just let him know that I love him, that the doctor says surgery was a total success, and that he's going to be fine. I realize the last time I shared a hospital with Sam was the day he was born, the day my life changed forever, the day I realized what it meant to be a parent, and to have the responsibility and joy of another soul's life entrusted to me. I was thirty. He will always be my baby boy.

Sitting here, I think about what an incredible man my son has become. For his whole life, he has stood by and waited to meet his little brother. Every year, with every intervention, we would optimistically tell Sam, "We're going to get him back." Sam would dutifully nod, but it never happened. He's had to shoulder his own grief about his brother, about the lost relationship through all of his childhood. With each conversation about Jamie these last few weeks, I've heard the emotion in Sam's voice, he's been hanging on every word, every story about what Jamie spelled. I accept that I can never fully understand what it's like to be Jamie's sibling, but I don't know how you do it with more patience and love than Sam has.

For many years, Sam volunteered at Victory, and many teachers would share stories with me about how warm, accepting, and easy-going he was with all the kids. When he was a high school senior, Sammy brought the house down at Victory's annual fundraiser, speaking eloquently before a crowd of more than 300 adults and letting his emotions show when he talked about Jamie. I've had so many people tell me how much Sam's speech moved them. As I process these thoughts and stare at Sam with all these needles and wires coming out of him, it's simply too much. The profound relief that Sam will make it and be OK. The rollercoaster of Jamie's emergence. The extreme stress of the last few hours. How can I be having my best life and worst all at once? I put my head in my hands, take a giant breath, and just let the tears flow. Shoulder-heaving sobs. Sammy stirs in his drugged-up haze. He grabs my hand and mumbles, "It's all good, pops. It's all good."

Philadelphia

*If you do not expect the unexpected you will not
find it, for it is not to be reached by search or trail.*

—Heraclitus

It's been three days since Sam's emergency surgery. The gravity of his circumstances, how close he came to the edge, it's hard to process right now. My family has basically taken over the Inn at Penn. Lisa and Quinny got here as soon as they could, my dad and sister Laura are still here, and our beloved nanny, Jordan, has also come out. We've been on a 24-hour vigil at Sam's bedside, each of the adults taking shifts, while we work to keep Quinny and Jamie both entertained and calm. The great news is that Sam's surgery was a success. They had to remove 100 percent of his spleen, but they found no damage to other organs, a huge risk when you lose as much blood as Sam apparently did. His surgeon, Dr. Brian Smith, has become the hero to our whole family, and we lavish him with gratitude every time he comes by to check on Sam.

Of course, I had to cancel the meetings Jamie and I were going to have in SoCal, and it's really unfortunate right now, because I can only guess how Jamie is feeling. The poor kid, he bore witness to the entire ordeal with Sam, including riding in the ambulance. I know he heard every word the doctors told me, and I'm also sure he picked up on the high tension in the room as various doctors rushed to keep Sam's vitals from crashing. I wish we could fly DM out for an emergency conversation, to let Jamie express himself. It's a bit torturous, and I just have to tell myself it's only a matter of time before Jamie is also open with us.

It's Tuesday evening, and Quinny is watching back-to-back *Shark Tank* episodes in our hotel room and seems to have fallen in love with the show. Perhaps she's our future capitalist. I'm sitting with Jamie and trying to occupy his time. He's been listening to music on his iPod with headphones, which is something he really only does when we travel. We've been spending a lot of time on the 26-letter stencil going through lessons, and I'm definitely feeling more confident as his communication partner. On a whim, I decide to ask Jamie a simple question, "Jamie, is there other music you would like to have on your iPod?" To date, we've had a pretty simple system for identifying music Jamie loves: if something comes on the radio when we're driving and he says, "Turn it up," that means he likes it and we add it to his playlist. I remember how DM got to an open place with Jamie by asking him something "low-risk," because if he is unable to spell on his own, I can just give him names of songs I know he loves for him to spell. It's worth a try.

Jamie smiles at me and, unprompted, spells, "T-U-P-A-C." I try to contain my excitement. "Anyone else?" Of course, he spells, "N-O-T-O-R-I-O-U-S-B-I-G." He already has a lot of Biggie's music on his playlist, so I ask, "Is there a song you really want?" Jamie spells, "Hypnotize." I'm floored and so jacked. It feels ridiculously glorious to be communicating with Jamie so directly that I never want it to end.

It seems Jamie doesn't want it to end, either. Over the next forty-five minutes, he spells a litany of artists and songs so vast and random that at times he's even stumping me, a music aficionado. He spells a Kyle Minogue song he really wants, Genuine, Fall Out Boy, Incubus, Limp Bizkit, Porno for Pyros, Eminem, Sia, Violent Femmes, and, a group so obscure for me that it took me awhile to believe what he was spelling, "Los Originales de San Juan." Every moment of spelling with Jamie is a joy. I no longer know the word I'm asking him to spell, I'm just sitting there being his vocal typewriter, and getting to know my son.

Lisa returns late from her shift watching Sam. It's after 11 p.m., and tonight my dad has the late shift. I will be relieving him around five in the morning. She's stressed. Sam has been having some postsurgery complications, and his bowels are in severe pain. The doctor has assured us this is normal, but after three days of being on adrenaline and no sleep, she's fried and a little discouraged. Of course, Jamie picks up on her mood and hears her concerning report. While we're engaged in conversation, I hear a familiar sound of moaning that Jamie does when he tantrums, and I turn to see him biting his arm extra hard while stomping. I intervene to stop him from hurting himself, grab his board, sit him down, and say, "Tell me what's happening."

Lisa stands there stunned as she watches Jamie spell, "I don't want Sam to die." My beautiful son, feeling pain and stress like all of us, is finally able to tell us what's going on. He's still amped up, and motions for the board. "I wrote Sam a note, and then he got injured." My God, the poor kid. He thinks somehow he had something to do with this. Brutal. We're able to spend the next twenty minutes walking Jamie through exactly what's going on with Sam, exactly what the doctors have told us, and reassure him that, no, his brother's life is not in danger and, no, his note didn't cause anything. Jamie spells, "I feel better now."

Thursday arrives, five days after Sam's injury, and things are getting better. Sam is cracking jokes again, and the daily visits from teammates are lifting his spirits. Seeing six teammates help Sammy do laps around the hospital floor hallway in his hospital gown and industrial socks is a sight to behold. It's also freed me up to schedule something I wasn't sure I would feel comfortable doing: taking Jamie to meet Honey, the amazing mom who opened this door for us, and her son Vince in person. It turns out they live just outside of Philadelphia, and the clinic that gave Vince the ability to use the letterboard—Inside Voice—is only a twenty-minute car ride away. Tom Foti, who runs the clinic, has agreed to have a lesson with Jamie and then facilitate a two-way lesson with Vince—and Jamie is clearly fired up.

My sister Laura wants to come along for the ride. Lisa and my dad can easily handle Sammy, so, after a quick breakfast, we head off into the suburbs of Philadelphia. My sister, eighteen months older, has always been a reliable friend and has always had my back. In high school, I was a bit sassy toward the older bullies, and Laura, a no-bullshit mother hen two grades above me, kept the bullies at bay. "Don't mess with my bro" was a common refrain.

Jamie has presented Laura with a new challenge. Ironically, her full-time job is an early childhood special education teacher in Northern Virginia, working with pre-K children on the spectrum. What Jamie is doing goes against everything she thought she knew about autism, and she has devoured all the video-taped sessions of Jamie spelling with EV and DM. There's now more than thirty hours of evidence. To her credit, she's diving in to learn and is extremely open to this new paradigm, but she wasn't ready for seeing Jamie spell in person. No one really is.

Tom Foti welcomes us into the nondescript offices of Inside Voice. Like many, he got into S2C for personal reasons. In this case, it was his older brother Brian who showed him the light, and Tom is now one of the community's most visible proponents, and he and his brother can be found at many conferences communicating together and advocating for nonspeakers and for letterboarding. The plan for today is that we will have an hour with Tom in the morning, break for lunch, and then meet Honey and Vince for an afternoon session. Jamie is notably excited as he sits down with Tom. Laura and I scurry into the back of the room. The opening lesson is about a band, Judah and the Lion, that I've never heard of. I'm struck by how quickly and smoothly Jamie is able to spell with Tom, and how consistent the methodology appears to be between Tom, DM, and EV. Jamie easily spells words like "Formula," "Puree," and "Twenty One Pilots." Before long, Tom is asking Jamie open questions, and he doesn't disappoint.

"What's your definition of 'eclectic'?" Tom inquires. "It is inspired by many elements," Jamie spells, and I hear a quick sniffle from Laura. Tom asks Jamie about the song "NAME," one of the band's more popular. "How do you think people could use this song in their everyday lives?" Jamie jumps right in:

"My interpretation on it is to savor the little moments so they may carry the darkest moments away. Thanks to my awesome circle I can now share in these moments." My tears are flowing, and I can feel Laura heaving next to me. I grab her hand. You can never un-see this.

Our quick lunch at Chipotle is filled with nervous anticipation, knowing that Honey and Vince will soon be on the scene. Laura explains how despite watching all the video, seeing her nephew spell in person has already changed her. She says she wants to learn how to do this, that her kids could benefit greatly.

Tom chooses a lesson for the group session about therapy dogs in Florida called the "K Ninth Circuit Program." The greeting with Honey and Vince was emotional, and we're now huddled together in a bigger room, with Jamie and Vince on opposite sides of a big conference table. Tom will be the moderator, working back and forth between Jamie and Vince with the letterboard. He's standing at a giant easel with a huge pad of paper on it, and I'm simply overwhelmed by the gravity of the moment, and the speed with which Jamie has made it to this moment. I can see he's feeling nervous and desperate to show Honey and Vince that he has maximized the life-changing opportunity they gave him.

Vince is sweet, kind, and warm. A bit older than Jamie, the deep introspection that I saw in the original texts sent by Honey still evident. The lesson explains how these therapy dogs are used in Florida to help children involved in the court system. Tom asks both boys, "What do you think about including adults in this program. Vince responds first, "I think it's crucial to not forget adults may need help, too." Jamie then chimes in, "I could not agree more. I can attest to it because I saw how much my parents struggled this week." Gulp. Done. Tears flowing. What a beautiful kid. Well, two beautiful kids, actually.

We're getting to the end of the lesson. Jamie and Vince have showered each other with "great point" and "I agree with Jamie" and "well said." Tom asks the boys, "Can you name a program you'd establish to help others?"

Jamie goes first, "I think what you're doing can take that spot, it's this method."

Vince has the last word and ends our amazing day in the perfect way, "That's my idea, too. The nonspeakers now have a voice."

We take pictures, more hugs, and then, Laura, Jamie, and I head back to Philly, where only more good news of Sam's recovery awaits. Sam will be able to check out of the hospital and stay with us in the hotel, and by Saturday we are cleared to fly—we're heading home.

Wilsonville

*If you accept the expectations of others, especially
negative ones, then you never will change the
outcome.*

—Michael Jordan

Victory Academy is housed in a beautiful, all-white, modern-barn building in the farmlands of Wilsonville, a 30-minute drive from our house. Parents move here from all over the country so their children can go to Victory. Roughly seventy-five students aged six to twenty with autism call Victory home, and we've always been grateful Jamie has Victory in his life. That is, until he could talk.

Right now, it's early March, and I'm sitting in the office of Tricia and Thea, Victory's cofounders, because I've asked for a meeting with one of Jamie's head teachers.

To put this meeting in proper context, some background is needed. When we first started taking Jamie down to DM and getting all these amazing words, we would share the news widely with teachers at the school in Jamie's orbit. In some cases, we'd get back the kind of reactions that we thought fit the moment, things like, "Oh My God! What a miracle! I'm crying!" Those same teachers were typically supercurious about S2C and would express an interest in learning more. Tricia and Thea, to their credit, were in that group as well, and after seeing video of Jamie for themselves, they started corresponding directly with EV about staff training, perhaps having her come out to the school, etc. With nearly one-third of Victory students being nonspeakers, this could obviously benefit many of the kids.

But then the BCBAs got involved (more on them in a moment). Lisa smelled the rat first. Some of the teachers on all the text chains we were sharing, who taught Jamie directly in his classroom, would only respond occasionally to our shared texts, and then with the most oddly unenthusiastic replies. Things like, "That's really nice for your family." Or, "It's so great when a child finds his voice." Wait a minute, what?

A little background: Victory has never seen anything like the miracle of Jamie at their school. Never, ever, never, ever. He was in a life skills class. They had no idea how smart he was. All those ideals that EV has about "presuming competence"? No, not in Jamie's class. To respond with anything short of acknowledging the torrential miracle that this really was caused us extreme confusion. Lisa put it best: "What the fuck is wrong with these people?"

EV had actually warned me about this. I think I just never believed it could happen at our beloved school. For background, "BCBA" means board certified behavior analyst, and it's the peak certification a teacher can get who works with children with autism. At Victory, it's almost half the faculty, and it's no small effort to become certified. BCBAs are experts in a form of autism therapy known as "ABA," which stands for Applied Behavior Analysis. It's a data-driven, rewards-based system for working with children with autism, but it also comes with its own share of controversy, because many people with autism consider ABA to be a cruel form of behavior modification with a faulty premise. In their opinion, autism is not a behavioral disability, and ABA presumes that most, if not all, children with autism are cognitively impaired. And, given everything I have seen with Jamie, I couldn't agree more with the critics.

BCBAs are always quick to cite "the research," and they tend to talk as if their way of teaching kids with autism were the only legitimate way, because it's based on science. To be honest, I didn't know or care much about this whole controversy. Victory claims to use a modified form of ABA that left many of the more controversial parts of ABA on the sidelines, and what I've generally seen at school is caring teachers who love my son and try hard to reach him.

What Jamie is now doing on the letterboard flies in the face of everything BCBAs are taught to believe. They're taught that kids like Jamie who are nonspeakers need ABA to help them navigate the world. The BCBAs answer for Jamie's miracle? It's not his words on the boards, it's the communication partner working with him. When I first heard this, I was astonished by how preposterous this was. It's a bit like telling my wife she didn't birth our three kids. Why even argue with someone who says or thinks something that ridiculous? Unfortunately, BCBAs carry a lot of weight in the autism world, and so their point of view, no matter how ignorant, can actually damage the credibility of S2C. I could write three books explaining to you how crazy this idea really is or tell you to watch the fifty-some hours of Jamie's S2C lessons we have on video, but I won't. I will just share this simple fact: Jamie spelled things with DM about his life that she didn't know. Enough said.

Tricia was incredibly enthusiastic about S2C from the start and everything Jamie is doing. She even sat in on one of Jamie's spelling sessions to see things for herself. She was in tears, as is anyone who knows Jamie and then sees him on the board for the first time—like Laura in Philadelphia, or my dad in Oceanside, or me in Virginia. We consider Tricia an ally, but she's let us know that the blowback from the BCBAs has been severe. Apparently, working with a child and a letterboard is actually grounds for decertification by the governing board of BCBAs, and Tricia has been managing a minirevolt behind the scenes. We don't have many details, but Tricia has explained to us, "I can't have over half my teachers leave en masse, but we will find a way through this." Tricia is one of the good people, and I can appreciate that she's in a tough spot, but if you take even one step back, this feels insane. Doesn't the school exist to help children find their voice and communicate with the world?

We came back from Philadelphia two weeks ago and brought Sam with us. He's still a few weeks from returning to school, and his season is clearly over. The great news is that he's maintained a great attitude and his recovery is on pace. We are counting our blessings and trying not to dwell on how dire his situation was.

Meanwhile, the connection Jamie and I established in Philly has only gotten better, and I am simply thrilled to report that I can communicate with my son anytime day or night. While the ridiculousness we are dealing with at this school is annoying, nothing can shake the joy ride we are on getting to know our son. I've also been sharing our story with many of my close autism friends around the country, and, to my delight and Jamie's, several have jumped into S2C including a good friend from Minneapolis who immediately called Growing Kids and booked her appointment. I asked Jamie if he would write a note to her son, Cade, and he was happy to help:

Dear Cade,

You will understand how this all works very soon. Hang in there and have fun. I hope you meet Dawnmarie soon. Only some parents have the courage to try this.

Tonight, I am able to write this because my parents took me to meet Elizabeth.

Jamie

Luckily, we have also developed a relationship with a talented and energetic local S2C practitioner—Dana Woodhouse—here in Portland. Dana is a newer practitioner, having successfully achieved fluency with her own son, Ethan. She's part of a growing second-generation network of teachers that EV is trying to train and certify all over the country through a newly created organization called the International Association of Spelling to Communicate, or "I-ASC," to make S2C accessible to more and more kids. Jamie has had a handful of sessions with Dana in Portland, and, to our delight, he was instantly able to be fluent and open with her, as well.

We've also gotten to know just how miserable Jamie has been at Victory for the last few years. Remember how I mentioned Jamie was having big issues at school where he would tantrum and then hit himself on the head? According to Jamie, "I was feeling very frustrated because [Jamie's previous teacher] was treating me like a retard." I ask him, "Was she mean to you?" He says, "Yes."

Now, seven months into the school year, the world has been turned upside down, and we're waiting for Victory to catch up so Jamie can use his letterboard at school and be in a more academic class that matches his intellectual level, which we're not even sure how to measure, but it's feeling more vast by the day. Or so we thought. That's all in doubt now, given the drama with the BCBAs. We're fine—we have a fluent Jamie on the boards. We have our son and the ability to really know him for the first time. We'd like the school to accommodate him, but if they don't, we will find another way. We're never going back to life before the letterboard.

Yesterday, Jamie came home from school, and he seemed anxious. I asked him how his day was, and he told me, "Boring." I said, "Do you want to stay at Victory?" He responded, "Yes. I need it to be OK to use the board. [My teacher] is not a believer." I ask him how he knows she isn't, and he says, "She asks questions that tell me she's a doubter." I ask him to give me an example. "Why is it your words if you can't say it?" he responds. I ask Jamie, "She said that to you?" as a I feel the anger bubbling up. "Yes," he responds.

Jesus. This kid. As if life hasn't been hard enough. He finally has a voice, and the very people supposed to be embracing this and teaching him . . . they are doubting him? Incomprehensible. I ask Jamie how it made him feel when he heard that.

"I felt so rageful. I am not sure my mind has let me internalize it." So now you know why we're having this meeting.

Oh, and one other thing. You see, when Jamie became fluent with me, we felt it was our moral duty to share our story with other families of nonspeaking kids in Jamie's class. There are quite a few. Jamie felt very strongly that it needed to be done. So, we did. And, understandably, some reached out to BCBA teachers to get their perspective. They advised against it. Actively against it. In fact, I later learned that a speech language pathologist, commonly known as an SLP, also called all the families of nonspeakers and actually told the parents S2C was not only harmful, but would cause their children to regress. Seriously.

I get right to the point, I'm the one who asked for this meeting. I explain to Jamie's head teacher that it's simply crucial that she believe in Jamie, and that he know it, too. At present, he doesn't believe she has faith in him, that she doesn't believe his words are real. I share exactly what he told me she said about him, and she denies it, saying it never happened. So, I ask her the question I've really wanted to know the answer to, the one that has mystified me from the first oddly unenthusiastic text response to all my reports of Jamie's miracle, "Do you believe it's Jamie's words coming out of the boards? We've shared with you all the video. He's now fluent with four different people (me, Dana, DM, Tom). Do you think it's him, or are we all skilled ventriloquists?" There's emotion in my voice and Jamie's teacher looks extremely uncomfortable, on the verge of tears. Tricia and Thea are riveted, awaiting a response. It comes out slowly, "I . . . don't . . . know."

Portland

Happiness radiates like the fragrance from a
flower and draws all good things towards you.
　　　　　　　　　　　　　—Maharishi Mahesh Yogi

It's mid-April. Like the rest of the country, we're on "lock-down" here in Oregon, which means the schools are closed and we're all home. Poor Sam, he was recovered from injury and ready to go back to college when everything shut down, so he's here for the duration. Jamie broke my heart to smithereens when he told me he "hopes Sam will be happy here." He loves his big brother so much and wants him to stay forever.

While the world feels a little nuts right now, Jamie's life is on absolute fire, and although we'd still love to be taking trips down to see DM, the truth is Jamie can talk with me on the board at such a clip that we are filling up notebooks with his beautiful words. Just this morning, he told me, "I have never felt happiness like this before." It really is that good—life is as close to unicorns and rainbows as it's ever been.

Importantly, Tricia has delivered the goods for Jamie in the greatest of ways. I knew she was the real deal, and she over-rode all the internal noise and has put Jamie in the right academic class at Victory with his new teacher, Cindy, who is not a BCBA and appears to be Jamie's biggest fan. Right before the lockdown, Cindy started to tutor Jamie one-on-one in math, and she got to not only see Jamie in action on the board, but he's proven to be extremely adept at math, and they are already deep into high school algebra. Jamie doesn't ever get problems wrong, and the truth is we have no idea what Jamie's outer bounds of math knowledge and ability might be, since before S2C they were only teaching Jamie rudimentary math. If you'd asked me back then if I thought Jamie could add, I would have said, "No." It's really painful to write that, but it's the truth. Cindy also let me know that she thought the controversy around Jamie's board was absurd, and that the whole reason she started working at Victory is the willingness of the school to try new things to help kids. Lisa and I love this woman, and so does Jamie.

Doing school virtually has provided for a natural transition to Jamie's new academic life, and Jamie's days are now filled with deep, enriching Zoom classes covering the following topics: Math, Social Studies, Science, Recreation, Transition, and then an even more advanced Math class with a wonderful teacher—also not a BCBA—named Johnny. Speaking of BCBAs and the whole process of ABA therapy, Jamie and I discussed the topic recently, and here's what he said: "I don't like ABA because it's cruel, they treat you like a stupid person. It's hard to like ABA because it doesn't presume competence. I think the teachers who do ABA are mean-spirited." Ouch. And, wow, this kid has a gift for forceful language.

Another unexpectedly wonderful aspect of these new Zoom classes is how much the other students have embraced Jamie. These beautiful kids, who've all had to face adversity and judgment from the wider world, cheer for Jamie when he gets the right answer, compliment him, and include him in all discussions. It's beautiful to watch. And then there's the teachers. Tricia has deftly managed Jamie's schedule to avoid the BCBAs, who still deem his board to be some sort of kryptonite, but that's actually left us with this amazing group of open-minded educators who all treat Jamie like the brilliant person he is. And, except for Cindy who experienced the letterboard before the lockdown, these Zoom classes are their first time seeing a child with autism on a board, and they have all been deeply moved, like anyone with a soul would be. It's incredible to witness.

Cora has emerged as one of Jamie's favorites. She teaches Outdoors & Recreation, which seems like a particularly tough place to be for virtual school, but she makes the most of it. She takes Jamie on virtual fieldtrips to parks throughout Oregon, helping us generate a list of future trips to take, and she's pushing Jamie to define which hobbies he's really interested in pursuing. She takes him through an extensive list of possible activities, and after much back and forth, two have emerged as winners: bicycling and kayaking.

Jamie tells Cora, "I want to have my own bike." For years, Jamie and I have ridden a tandem bike all over Portland. During the lockdown, it's been a daily event. Of course, he's ready to be his own man—he's in his late teens! Jamie, with Cora's help, also makes it clear that two-wheeled bikes are hard for him to manage. He's very scared he will fall. Cora does the research and proposes an adult trike bike with three wheels, two in the back. "Yes, that's what I want" is Jamie's clear response.

Honestly, it's a bittersweet moment for me. Biking has always been one of our things, and the tandem has made it a very personal experience for us. Can he really handle his own bike? So many decisions to make when you are the navigator, so many risks. Is he really ready? And am I ready? My son, who I always thought would be dependent, is flexing his independence.

With some pain in the heart, I order the bike from Rose City Bikes. They tell me it's backordered a couple of weeks, which will give me a little time to prepare to let go.

Sisters, Oregon

While we try to teach our children all about life,
our children teach us what life is all about.
—Angela Schwindt

Central Oregon is breathtakingly beautiful, and it's an extra-warm day here for mid-May. We've escaped Portland for the weekend, where things feel somewhat oppressive, and it's great to be in a place that seems indifferent to and insulated from the daily news. We're here for a specific reason: after four long weeks, THE bike has arrived. Jamie's bike, an adult trike from Sun Bicycles. And he is fired up. Last night he told me, "I am very excited." I asked him if he felt ready to navigate everything himself on the bike, and his simple answer was "Yes." Lisa starts micromanaging the littlest details of Jamie's ride. He spells, "Mom is bothering me." She relents.

Jamie has been blowing our minds now with regularity. The most recent event? Calculus. Dana introduced us a few weeks ago to Vaishnavi Sarathy—we call her "Vaish"—a chemistry PhD who tutors kids like Jamie. Not only is she comfortable working with the letterboard, but she knows exactly how smart nonspeakers really are and, after a quick diagnostic, deems Jamie fully ready to tackle calculus. It's humbling to think about how much we underestimated Jamie. Our first session was surreal. Lisa and I attended together and sat back and watched

Vaish take Jamie through complex mathematical concepts that two Stanford grads couldn't remember or solve. "We're going to need to find a college professor to work with Jamie soon," Vaish tells us, "he's going to tap out my knowledge within a few lessons." Vaish's own son Sid, who has Down syndrome, also uses a letterboard to communicate. Physics and chemistry are next.

We're staying here in a beautiful community called Black Butte Ranch. We're regulars, and the place is filled with relatively flat bike paths and far less traffic than in Portland. It feels like a great place for Jamie to be more independent. It's clear Jamie is yearning to draw firmer boundaries and flex his independence. At the same time, he has seventeen years of habits to break. We've been making sure, every day, to remind Jamie that he is in charge of his future, his needs. Last night, I was working on this concept with Jamie, and after listening to me emphasize that only he can choose what he wants, he quickly spelled, "I'd like pancakes for breakfast every day." That felt like progress!

It's been almost three months since Jamie and I first became fluent together in Philadelphia, and the lockdown has allowed us to have months of unexpected time with Sam, who is now fully recovered and back to his old self. He works out often, and I can see the drive that made him a great athlete in the first place re-emerge. He now has something to prove.

Another amazing development, organized by our local S2C practitioner Dana, is a weekly Zoom-based call that's been named "Dude-Bro Social." Jamie, Ethan, Finley, Liam, and Evan, five beautiful teenagers all using letterboards, are now meeting every week to discuss whatever topics they want. In each case, a parent serves as communication partner, and the boys do their best to pretend we aren't there and focus on one another. Teen slang abounds. They discuss girls, a recent divorce, school stress, the lockdown, favorite music, hobbies, future goals—the list is endless.

One teen asks his buds if they have any advice for how he can move a relationship with a girl to the next level. Jamie jumps in to provide advice. "I think you should ask her to go on a walk on the beach. You can offer to take her to a movie, too. You need to go for it, life is short." I wish I could share more, but what happens in Dude-Bro stays in Dude-Bro. It's their time, and it's a ridiculous honor to bear witness. After several weeks, Jamie tells me, "I feel closest to other letterboarders."

Earlier this week, something unexpected happened. A study was published by three professors from the University of Virginia in the journal *Nature* titled "Eye-Tracking reveals agency in assisted autistic communication." It affirms what Lisa and I already know: that letterboarders are spelling their own words. The authors concluded, "the speed, accuracy, timing, and visual fixation patterns suggest that participants pointed to letters they selected themselves, not letters they were directed to by the assistant." My reaction to the study? "Yeah, no shit." But I know these studies need to happen to get the denialists and haters to stop doubting kids like Jamie, and I forward it to Tricia. I'm sure all the BCBAs will remain skeptical because it threatens their worldview. In Part IV, I will address some of this controversy in more detail.

Right now, I'm focused on Jamie. For years, I've taken him on a pretty extensive daily tandem bike ride here at Black Butte, but it feels a little long for Jamie to be doing all by himself. There are a few roads to cross, and there will be oncoming bike traffic and pedestrians—a ton of separate decisions to make, all while Jamie needs to be getting used to both hand brakes and steering. I ask Jamie if he'd like to start with a simple, shorter ride. "No, I want to do the regular ride," he tells me. Deep breath, and I can only say, "Okay, bud. Let's go."

And the bike ride turns out to be one of the more intensely beautiful experiences of my life. Jamie leads the whole way. He knows the route, and he has zero problem on the bike. Steering and braking is, inexplicably, perfect. He moves where he needs to move on the paths to manage oncoming traffic, slows down on the bigger downhills, and digs in deep to climb the bigger hills. I'm riding behind him, shouting words of encouragement, but he hardly needs them. He's sitting up straight, completely in command of his bike. The whole ride takes us more than forty-five minutes, and he's perfect, from start to finish. Perfect. I'm a little stunned and realize I'm doing something that's been done to Jamie his whole life. I'm reminded of a lesson I did with him on Albert Einstein. At the end, I asked him if he related at all to Einstein? "Yes, because I was underestimated."

The guilt can show up at times like this, too, when I should just be celebrating. How in the hell did I miss this? How did I miss this brilliant boy and let him suffer in silence for so long? The single biggest error I made was that I considered whatever words came out of Jamie's mouth to be reflective of his cognition. If his most complex sentence was "Potty please," then that's where he was on the IQ scale. Of course, this could not have been more wrong. Rationally, I get it. I know I was doing my best as a parent and that everyone missed Jamie. Most people who interacted with Jamie had the best of intentions, but we all missed it. I still feel awful about it sometimes. And then I remind myself that it could still be six months ago, it could still be the time before we went to Herndon, and I shudder and thank God that we're here.

I asked Jamie a follow-up question after that Einstein lesson. After he told me that he related to Einstein and how everyone underestimated him, I asked Jamie if he was mad at Mom and Dad because we underestimated him, and he gave an answer that I am starting to realize is a very Jamie thing to say because Jamie has more grace than anyone I have ever met. Here's what he said: "No, because you never gave up on me."

Lake Oswego

I'm still down with my homies from the home-
town, and if you need, need anything at all
I drop it all for y'all, if my homies call.

—Tupac Shakur

It's the last day of July, over 90 degrees, and Jamie and I are paddling on Lake Oswego, a beautiful lake just south of Portland. It's after 6 p.m. but still very hot, which is rare for the Pacific Northwest. Thanks to Cora, we're riding a tandem kayak, which Jamie had identified during that Zoom meeting with her as another activity he'd be really interested in trying. The kayak arrived two weeks ago, and we've been out on the lake almost every day. It made me so happy when he spelled, "I love being in nature and being on the water."

In early July, Victory was able to start in-person summer school with some modest restrictions due to the coronavirus. Mercifully, Jamie's day goes from 12:30 to 4:30 p.m., which means he's been able to maintain summer sleeping hours. For Jamie, returning to Victory has been an incredible roller coaster of emotions. On his first day back, we asked him how his day had gone, and he explained, "It was the best day of my life at Victory." Keep in mind, not only was Jamie finally in the right classroom with his teacher Cindy and the wonderful kids he'd gotten to know on Zoom, but it was also the first time he ever had access to the letterboard at school outside of the handful of tutoring sessions he'd had with Cindy right before the lockdown. Presently, I am serving as his communication partner. Jamie, however, has made it clear that he would greatly prefer if his parents were not with him at school, so we are working with Dana to train two people to rotate being his communication partner come the fall.

One of the many amazing things that's been notable about Jamie's return to Victory has been the absence of behavioral issues. Before the letterboard, Jamie was deemed a behavioral problem, and there was a "flow chart" put together with all these convoluted metrics for Jamie to meet in order to regain various freedoms within the school. If he had two days in a row with no armbite, he could extend recess by twenty minutes, but if an arm bite happened before that, he'd be back on the yellow path and only get ten minutes and . . . it was confusing as hell, made no real sense, but was "rooted in ABA," whatever that means. We had plenty of spreadsheets and data given to us, and Jamie was miserable. Now that he can communicate? No issues. Go figure. S2C has done in six months what all those ABA charts and more than a decade of schooling didn't do.

I'm paddling in the back, and I've pulled up to a dock on a tiny little island called Schaeffer Island in the middle of the lake. Having the letterboard has created so many tiny changes for us, and it's hard to keep track. For example, I've packed Jamie's crocs for this ride because we're going to jump in the lake near the shore for a little swim, and Jamie informed me that he didn't like the slippery rocks on the bottom of the lake, so I have his shoes. He also told me he doesn't like swimming in the lake if he can't see the bottom, so this is a perfect spot because it's very shallow. These tiny accommodations add up to a much happier and much less frustrated kid, and we take the board everywhere we go. Wants and needs are met, and daily frustrations are quickly resolved. For years, I've been getting Jamie a chicken bowl at Chipotle. He let me know he prefers steak.

Still, returning to Victory has been hard on Jamie, because he sees his beloved former classmates, all of them nonspeakers, and it makes him both sad and angry. Last week, after a few days of Jamie explaining how frustrated he was, I asked him if he'd like to write a note to Tricia and Thea and tell them how he feels. He was quick to say, "Yes." Here's what he wrote (his former classroom is called "Cedar"):

Dear Tricia and Thea, I think the Cedar kids need to learn how to letterboard. I think it's not fair to have them in there not able to talk. Now is the time for action. I hope you agree and I have many ideas for how to help them. No one should be denied their voice. Sincerely, Jamie

As you can imagine, I was insanely proud of what Jamie wrote. But he took it a step further, when he demanded we meet with Tricia and Thea, and that he attend the meeting. He told me, "They need to hear from me directly." So, at the end of last week, we did just that, we arranged a meeting with Tricia and Thea. We asked Jamie if he might like to put some of his ideas down on paper before the meeting, and he said he would. Here are his suggestions:

I think Tricia needs to meet with all the Cedar parents.

I think the teachers in Cedar need to learn how to letterboard.

I think all the teachers at Victory need to learn about letterboarding.

I think Victory should have DM present to all the teachers.

I think some teachers should not be able to work with nonspeakers.

I think Tricia should make Cedar teachers not be able to warn parents against letterboarding.

I think the curriculum should reflect the motor challenges of the students.

I think Tricia should have EV come to the school and meet with the teachers.

As Jamie cranked out this list, Lisa and I were simply dumbfounded. Our sweet, gracious son is also a loyal friend and an activist. Our meeting with Tricia and Thea was very productive. Jamie truly bristles whenever I refer to what happened to him as "a miracle." He tells me, "All nonspeakers are capable of doing what I did." I ask him about his classmates. He tells me they can all "sense what each other are feeling" and that they are all exactly like him.

During the meeting, we took Tricia and Thea through Jamie's entire list, and they listened closely. We made the point, as forcefully as we could, that Jamie felt every nonspeaker at Victory could do exactly what he did, and that if Victory could endorse S2C that may impact the willingness of other parents to give this a try. At the end Jamie told Tricia, "You are doing a great job," and brought her to tears.

I could tell Jamie was a little unsatisfied with the meeting. Tricia was honest with him about the BCBAs and the roadblocks they create for adopting letterboards throughout the school. Of the half-dozen parents we personally approached about letterboarding back in February, two have started lessons, but that leaves four kids in Jamie's old class who he feels have been left behind, and perhaps a dozen kids in other classrooms who are either nonspeakers or unreliable speakers. He tells me he wants me to call their parents again and makes me promise to "never give up on any of my friends." Dutifully, I did just that, and one of the families took me up on the offer to come by this past weekend.

Phil, Jennifer, and their son Michael showed up on Saturday, after I explained to them that Jamie had insisted I invite them over. Right before they arrived, Jamie told me, "I'm a little nervous about Michael's parents. I so want them to help Michael, and I hope they listen." They were very polite and admitted that one of the BCBAs had talked them out of trying things back in February. Jamie was sitting attentively, listening to the conversation, when I noticed he wanted to say something. "I know Michael can do this. He's going to be great." Phil, the father, was immediately stunned as he watched Jamie spell for the first time. Jennifer, the mother, was an instant weepy mess. Jamie spells, "Everyone cries the first time they see this." It's true. You can't really explain what it's like to bear witness to a nonspeaker letterboarding. You just have to see it for yourself. I can tell that Phil is already sold. He engages in a back-and-forth with Jamie, and when I tell them that I genuinely believe Michael can do this, too, the tears flow. Just then, in the midst of Jamie thanking them for being willing to bring Michael to see him, Michael gets up and sits down next to Jamie on the couch for a closer look. Phil looks at his son and says, "Michael, do you want to try this?" Michael gives him an emphatic thumbs up, his sign word for "yes."

Jamie was also deadly serious about getting DM to meet with Victory. Earlier this week, we confirmed with her to come up here next month for four days to meet with Tricia and Thea and all the Victory teachers in Jamie's orbit (of course, none of the BCBAs will be there). Due to the length of her visit, we've also scheduled spelling lessons for Michael and the two other nonspeakers who are doing S2C. One of the other families has agreed to come visit a couple weekends from now. We won't stop until we've gotten every family to at least see Jamie for themselves, and I know Jamie will never give up.

We're about ninety minutes into the kayak ride, and the sun is starting to go down. This is my favorite time to be on the lake, and I love the solitude of being here with Jamie. He sits in front of me, and I spend most of our time talking to him about anything that's on my mind. I realize I have been using this time to try and freeze time for a moment and just appreciate the joy of life right now. Sam is all better. He'll be heading back to school in late August. Quinny is happy and healthy, and her life is filled with great friends and activity. She's emerging as a confident young woman. Lisa and I have never been happier, and the darkness has truly lifted.

Jamie's favorite teacher, Molly, has been in his life for the past decade. Early on, she was his classroom teacher, but for the past few years she's taken on the role of transition specialist at Victory, helping students think about life after high school. As much as we loved Molly, meeting with her about Jamie used to be superdepressing, because we were all sitting around the table trying to guess what he might want to do with his future. Now, the meetings with Molly are gold mines of new information, all of it generated by Jamie. Recently, he told Molly his ten-year goal was to be "talking and married." He wants to go to college. He wants to study neuroscience, with a focus on motor disabilities. Molly asked him what he might like to do for a job. To my stunned surprise he said, "I'd like to write a book with my dad." Molly replied, "Why would you like to do that?" Jamie spelled, "to inspire others like me." After we get off the call, Jamie has more to say. "I think we need to make a movie, too." I ask him why he thinks that's important. "Because seeing is believing. When people see me spell, they cry."

So, tonight is a special night. It's day one of Jamie writing his portion of the book. I told him I'd be happy to tell the story from my perspective, but the world is much more interested in hearing from him. He tells me he finds writing long-form prose a little daunting, as he's never done it before. He says he'd prefer I ask him questions and he answer them. Great, I'll do that. He also says he wants his buddies in Dude-Bro to have a chance to tell their story in the book, too. No problem.

I decide to open with some basic questions and see where it goes. "Jamie," I ask, "why write a book?" I anticipate the answer, but I still love seeing him spell it: "I want to inspire other non-speakers that they can do this."

"Why do you care so much about helping other people?" I inquire. "I feel strongly that everyone should have their own voice," he spells.

"How has your life changed since you started letterboarding?"

"I am able to share my feelings and dreams, it is the awesomest thing that has ever happened to me."

"How has it impacted your mood?"

"I am so much happier now than I used to be. Now I can share my feelings when I feel frustrated and it's so much better. I never get to the point of frustration that I used to get."

I tell Jamie he did a wonderful job, that he's done enough for tonight. I tell him that he humbles me with his grace, his grit, his warm heart, and his dedication. I tell him that I love him, and that he will be an inspiration for so many others like him.

In three weeks, Jamie will be eighteen. A year ago, we were preparing to file guardianship papers that would allow us to make all of Jamie's decisions for him. We no longer need those. Will he be married and talking in ten years? We dare not underestimate him—we made that mistake for way too long.

II

Q&A with Jamie

Jamie's Reaction to the Book

I wrote the narrative of Part I to completion and then shared it all with Jamie to get his reaction and input. What follows is the back-and-forth of our conversation as I read him each section.

Introduction, where I share hard feelings about Jamie's prospects
Jamie: I thought, "Oh my God, I didn't know how hard it was for you and Mom not to know what I was thinking. I feel like I made you too worried. I love to listen to this story."
J.B.: Did it make you feel guilty?
Jamie: No, I kept thinking that I wish I could have told you I was listening to everything and was sincerely smart.
J.B.: Would you like to say more?
Jamie: No, I'm good.

Vancouver, where I detail our trip to Canada to do a fecal microbial transplant
Jamie: Yes, I thought I wish you knew how much I understood. I was very excited about Canada because I knew it could help me. I wish you could have known.
J.B.: Do you think it helped?
Jamie: Yes, I think it made me more calm. It was an overall reduction in anxiety.

Portland, where I talk about an outburst Jamie had at school
Jamie: I kept thinking how much I hated going to Victory and how they treated me like I was stupid. Yes, I was miserable at school and really wanted to go home so you were right. To have to be treated that way every day not only made me mad but also made me very mad that you guys kept taking me there.

J.B.: I'm really, really sorry.

Jamie: Yes, I know you guys didn't know how bad it was. I want you to know that I'm not mad at you anymore.

J.B.: If you were, that would be very understandable.

Jamie: I know but I'm not.

J.B.: How would you describe your state of mind when you have these outbursts?

Jamie: I think it's like having a seizure.

J.B.: Do you remember the experience afterward?

Jamie: No, it's like I'm not even there.

J.B.: Can you tell when they're coming?

Jamie: Not always, sometimes it sneaks up on me.

J.B.: Do you have any advice for parents who have children who have these outbursts?

Jamie: I don't know, I would say find a way to communicate.

J.B.: We really never have these episodes anymore; why do you think that is?

Jamie: I think because I'm so much happier.

Oceanside, where I talk about sitting in the hot tub with Jamie and how my whole world was about to change for the better
Jamie: I felt that you must have known that something was about to change. I remember being there and I was really happy, it was a really fun weekend. Did you always feel that you would figure it out?

J.B.: Yes.

Jamie: That's what I thought.

Beaverton, where I detail getting the text and call from Honey
Jamie: I am so happy that Honey made that call to you. She is a wonderful person. I think we should put her in the movie—she is a wonderful spokesperson. Yes, I think that Honey saved my life. I think we need to thank her. I think she is an amazing person. I want her to be in the movie, I want Vince to be in the movie, too.

PDX, where I describe running into sportscaster Lamar Hurd at the airport and the generosity of parent Elizabeth Zielinski
Jamie: I loved hearing that. I remember that Lamar saw us at the airport. Yes, I think he was an omen, he is such a good person. I liked hearing about what Elizabeth said [that Jamie would be spelling open very soon]. She was right, she knew I could do it. I want you to thank her for me. I'm glad we saw Lamar.

Herndon, detailing Jamie's first S2C lesson with EV
Jamie: I was thinking about how much excitement I felt when Elizabeth told me I was smart. No one had ever said that to me. She opened the door for me to have my life again. She is the most adorable-est person in the world! Yes, thank you so much Elizabeth, I think you truly saved my life. You are a special person.
J.B.: Do you think EV is a heroic person?
Jamie: Yes, she is unique because she saw what others missed.
J.B.: She's sometimes attacked for her nontraditional views; what do you think of that?
Jamie: Yes, that is really sad, but I'm glad she never gives up.

Dulles Airport, detailing Day 2 with EV when he spelled "herbivore"

Jamie: I remember spelling "herbivore" and how shocked you were. It was a shock for me, too, because no one had ever believed in me like that before. Elizabeth surely knew I knew the answer, she is an amazing person.

J.B.: Tell me more about spelling "herbivore" and how you felt.

Jamie: I knew that I would never be the same.

Newport Beach, when Jamie first meets Dawn Marie Gaivin (DM)

Jamie: I loved getting to know more about your experience with DM. It was so awesome for me to be there with her. I think DM is the best teacher in the world, no one can teach me like she can. I think every nonspeaker can learn to spell if they work with DM. I remember asking if I would have to go back to three boards after I left, because I never wanted to go back. I loved being in California. It was perfect.

Palm Springs, providing more details about Jamie's time with DM, his big emotional cry, and his note to the president

Jamie: I loved hearing that, I'm so glad we went to Palm Springs. It was great to be there because I could sit in the sun and think about how my life was changing. I remember crying, and I was crying for all the times I couldn't talk about my feelings and how glad I was to be done with that. I think that weekend was when I knew that my life would never be the same.

College Park, providing more detail about our time with DM, highlighting Jamie's first note to his brother, Sam, and the first hint that Sam may have a serious injury

Jamie: I remember writing that note to Sam, not knowing what lay ahead. I felt great writing that to Sam. Now I think I might have played a role in his injury. No person should have to go through what Sam did. I'm always keeping a close eye on Sam whenever he plays.

JB: Your note had nothing to do with Sam's injury; it was just a coincidence. Do you believe me?

Jamie: I do rationally, but I can't help feeling that way sometimes.

Penn Presbyterian, providing the details on Sam's injury

Jamie: I get anxious just thinking about this. I'm so grateful for Dr. Smith, he saved Sam. I think Sam was very lucky to be in Philadelphia.

JB: You realize we were only there because I wanted Sam to see you spell?

Jamie: No, I hadn't thought about that.

JB: Well, how does it make you feel?

Jamie: I'm glad I helped make sure we were there.

Philadelphia, where Sam is improving, my sister Laura gets emotional watching Jamie spelling, and Jamie meets Vince and Honey for the first time

Jamie: I loved hearing about Laura being inspired by me. I remember being so nervous to spell with Vince. I believe Vince and his mom saved my life. I want you to thank them for telling us about S2C. They are special people. I think it's important for everyone who is letterboarding to share their story. I think you can tell if someone will believe you by how they react to your story. I think most people will listen. I hope most people will listen to us.

Wilsonville, where we experience conflict and disbelief from some of Jamie's teachers
JB: Jamie felt this section was too harsh because I named some teachers, so he had me go back and rewrite it and tone everything down. He said, "They meant well, they were just ignorant."

Portland, where Jamie works with his teacher Cora to identify his love for riding his own bike
Jamie: I am so grateful to Cora for helping me decide what I wanted. I think getting that bike has been one of my favorite moments, and I love riding it. I'm excited to hear more.

Sisters, where Jamie rides his new bike for the first time
Jamie: I remember that bike ride, I was so excited! I think that's when I really knew that things were really changing forever.

Lake Oswego, where Jamie has Michael come over, plans for a visit from DM, and begins to write this section of the book
Jamie: I loved that. I think that Michael is going to do great. I think that having DM come up sincerely impacted Victory. I think I'll be talking much sooner than ten years, I think I will be talking in six months. I am glad we wrote this book. I hope it inspires other nonspeakers. I'm feeling really good about it. I'm glad that we shared it with the world.

Additional Q&A with Jamie

The below is the transcript of a conversation between J.B. and Jamie.

J.B.: Tell me about life before you learned to letterboard.

Jamie: I would say it was like trying to talk but nothing would come out. It was very frustrating, and I often felt my life would always be this way.

J.B.: How were you able to find joy and remain sane when no one knew the real you?

Jamie: I kept believing that someday I would be able to talk and that kept me going.

J.B.: Did it consume your thoughts, this yearning to be able to express yourself?

Jamie: No, I just accepted that I couldn't control it.

J.B.: What's it like when you try to talk?

Jamie: It's hard. I don't feel like I can make the words come out of my mouth.

J.B.: Watching you spell on the letterboard, it seems easy. Is it?

Jamie: Yes, it's easy to spell this way.

J.B.: Did art or music help you in terms of having some sort of outlet for expression?

Jamie: I think music has always helped me.

J.B.: When you listen to music, do you sing the songs in your head?

Jamie: Yes, I do, I always have.

J.B.: Is there a favorite you love to sing?

Jamie: "Man in the Mirror."

J.B.: Are your childhood memories filled with thoughts of the frustration of not being able to talk?

Jamie: Yes, I have always been able to think like anyone else.

J.B.: Did you ever feel like life wasn't fair to you?

Jamie: No, I felt that I was lucky to have a family that always loved me. I felt that you guys would figure it out. [Dad takes a break to stem flow of tears.]

J.B.: Your frustration at school seemed to grow. Is that true?

Jamie: Yes, it's sucked for years. I was so sick of being treated like someone who was stupid.

J.B.: I'm so sorry, bud. I never would've made you go if I knew that.

Jamie: I know you meant well.

J.B.: You mentioned that ABA therapy was really hard for you, that you didn't like its rigidity. Can you say more?

Jamie: Other than on task behavior, everything is seen as stimming. Children move their bodies a lot; however, only autistic children get in trouble for moving.

J.B.: Do you know I always have your back?

Jamie: Yes, I meant it when I said you are my ride or die homie.

J.B.: What do you imagine doing in the future?

Jamie: College. Then, I think it would be nice to spend time in a lab doing research. I want to research the brain and motor connection.

J.B.: Tell me about math.

Jamie: Math makes me right-minded in ways that make my brain happy. I get numbers like hearing my name makes me feel. My mind has no idea why numbers are so easy.

J.B.: Does money matter to you?

Jamie: I don't care about money. I care about my family and my friends.

J.B.: Your great friend from Victory, Shane, is finally working with the letterboard. How does that make you feel?

Jamie: I hope he has mad love for the letterboard.

J.B.: What makes you happiest right now?

Jamie: I'm so happy I can talk to my family about everything.

J.B.: You've explained how it's hard for you to speak; are there other challenges you experience with motor planning?

Jamie: I think it's hard for me to get my body to move how I want.

J.B.: A year ago we had never heard of S2C. What are your first thoughts now when you wake up in the morning?

Jamie: I'm grateful for the life I have and excited for where it's going.

J.B.: We have learned you have an incredible capacity to retain and analyze information, do math, and listen intently. Are there other unique gifts you think you have?

Jamie: Yes, I do. I think I may be uniquely able to read people like a savant. Variety is my specialty, I think I'm good at many things.

J.B.: Do you have a sense of how smart you are?

Jamie: I think I am smarter than most people.

J.B.: You sometimes wave your arms in the air or rock side to side. What can you tell us about those movements that would help others understand you better?

Jamie: I use those movements to help me stay calm.

J.B.: You have been incredibly forgiving toward everyone who underestimated you for all these years. How are you able to be so gracious?

Jamie: I think everyone was doing their best, and I know you love me.

J.B.: Are there any personality traits you think nonspeakers have in common?

Jamie: I think all the spellers are much more likely to be kind and forgiving toward others and are the most vastly nice people in the world. I think spellers are very loving and care about others.

J.B.: What's school been like with the board and with Cindy? How have the other kids in your class treated you?

Jamie: It's awesome, everyone has been great.

J.B.: How were you able to teach yourself to read, spell, and do math?

Jamie: I think how I did it will remain unknown because I have no idea.

J.B.: What was it like to have people talk about you in your presence before you could speak?

Jamie: It was really frustrating, I felt like talking but couldn't, no way I ever want to be there again.

J.B.: What is the one thing you would like someone first meeting you to know?

Jamie: I'm smart and I understand everything.

J.B.: What do you feel you have missed out on the most in your first seventeen years?

Jamie: I wish I had the chance to make more friends.

J.B.: Are there silver linings or blessings to what you have had to endure?

Jamie: Yes, I think I have had to learn to be resilient.

J.B.: What is the best way for people to connect or interact with you socially?

Jamie: I would say express yourself because I can understand you.

J.B.: Is there a way we can help you deepen your relationship with your siblings?

Jamie: I think you can help me have conversations.

J.B.: What has it been like for your extended family to learn how smart you really are?

Jamie: It's been amazing to have everyone know the truth. I'm so happy they know.

J.B.: Is there one thing that you are most proud of so far in life?

Jamie: I think I'm most proud that I never allowed my disability to define me. I'm proud that I never gave up. I think I was born to do this and inspire others. I really want others to know that they can do this. I think my proudest accomplishment will be the people I inspire.

J.B.: Do you have a life philosophy?

Jamie: I think my philosophy is to make every day count because I have so much to do, I want to learn about everything in the world.

J.B.: What advice would you give a nonspeaker?

Jamie: I would tell them to try it. They can do it, and it will change their life.

III

Dude-Bro Speaks

I went thirty years without being able to commu-
nicate my deep thoughts. I am only now realizing
the magnitude of my potential lost through years
of being presumed incompetent. It is devastating.
Yet I am also full of hope.

—Danny Whitty

There are many extraordinary stories about nonspeakers who finally are blessed with the ability to communicate through S2C. In the case of Danny Whitty, it didn't happen until he was well past his thirtieth birthday. Last September, he published an extraordinary essay on the blog Medium.com titled "Listen for unspoken voices, our non-speaking views must be valued." Mr. Whitty is particularly concerned with advocating for the large portion of the autism community—estimates are roughly 40 percent—who are nonspeakers. He writes:

What we non-speaking autistics must do is get our unspoken voices heard. With communication aids like the letterboard or keyboard or whatever works for you, we should clamor for our rights. We should advocate for ourselves. We should make our experiences part of the mainstream autistic narrative.

What Mr. Whitty wrote rang very familiar to me, because I've had the distinct pleasure of sitting in on Jamie's weekly Zoom calls for his "Dude-Bro" social hour that I already talked about.

The need for nonspeakers to self-advocate is a common theme of discussion among the boys.

On several occasions, Jamie has brought up this book, and he decided he'd really like his buddies to join him by sharing their own comments and stories with the world. What follows are the thoughts and insights of five extraordinary young men— Ethan, Finley, Evan, Liam, and Vince—but first, a word from Jamie:

> I would like to introduce my amazing friends who inspire me every week with their great wisdom and compassion. I hope you enjoy hearing from the Dude-Bros!

Ethan, Age 19
Portland, Oregon

Health is not nutrition. Love is nutrition of a different meat. History dedicates others to tell the tale of some people yet it does not tell the story of the voiceless.

Let us tell the story not of those for whom more, not less, is heard. Talk not of those ready voices. Talk instead of those who live in darkness.

Respect only comes when others view you as having worth. I had no equity in silence. I needed to deposit my words in the perceptual bank of human connections. Only in this account do I own any collateral. This bothers me. Humans should bestow kindness in places they don't often travel. I shouldn't have to please you to get your respect.

To have my words I need my mind and motor in harmony. Help comes only in the form of a trained partner quietly following my lead and stemming the flow of motor loops that plague my neurology. You have no idea, none at all, the energy it takes to limit my loops. My motor is a mess of impulses easily and often hit by compulsions. Certain compulsions take over, getting in the way of doing anything else. Being stuck is an exhausting process. So many people think I want to do the things I do. Honestly, I hate stims. They make me look stupid. I am not stupid. My body is my limitation to accessing the world.

Sometimes I believe that my life began the day I met a teacher named Elizabeth [Vosseller]. Tart memories of listening, not speaking, were my life. Being called intellectually low hit my heart like a weight to the gut. The morning we met was sunny. I felt scared. Momma let me go in with my shirt off so I didn't run. We rounded the corner and I saw a certain teacher with long blonde hair. Would she like me? Would I cause her to be disgusted? To ready myself, I whistled. Yet she spoke to me with humor and some sort of respect. Yes, I thought, give her the whole show.

"You must not spit on me," she said. "We are here to learn a new way to communicate. You are smart but your body is another matter."

You must remember, I heard nothing but how I was so difficult. Teachers had long litanies of my deficits. Too much spitting, too much movement, too much foolish running. I could please no one. Elizabeth sees me. She does not care if I spit so long as I spell. She looks inside and sees who I want to be. One time I went under the table to hide and she went under too. Momma says Elizabeth sorted us out. She pushed us through to where we needed to be.

The lesson we learned that day was on Midas. He loved his gold so much he made it his only wish. He ended up turning his only daughter into gold. His most beloved object turned out not to be his gold but his child. He stopped desiring things of money and instead desired only his not-gold daughter.

The question I was asked was how did Midas feel when he turned his only child into gold? The easy word was sad. That was not my word. I knew what word I wanted. It was hard to make my hand move where I wanted. Just looking at the letter was challenging. I got agitated. I pushed and hit the board.

"Just relax," said Elizabeth. Her voice pulled me out of my agitation.

My word was DEVASTATED. I spelled it, letting myself relax. It was my word. I chose it. Someone else did not put it on an icon for me to choose. The difference is gray scale compared to technicolor. I never wanted to have my words picked out for me again.

Sorting out my mind is hard. This being I live in seems to please only itself. Then it eats my hopes and dreams. Quietly, Momma tries to find ways to help. She found Elizabeth. She promised not to unsee what she had seen. Working really hard, we made it happen. I find new ways to learn each day.

This week I learned what a black hole is; I learned about the event horizon. One can get into the event horizon but one can never get out. It is necessary to travel faster than the speed of light to escape. No one knows what it is to be beyond this border.

I do. It is where I lived before I learned to use a board to spell. I hereby leverage my words against your expectations of me.

Finley, Age 18
San Diego, California

Invite you to take a walk with me back in time. Seeing myself as hardened, misty, and muted. My inner child was hindered. He melted down a lot. He didn't have the inner wherewithal to cope with his limitations. Rinsing was required. He would maneuver right next to Mom's heart and Mom would heal him with her love. Sins were mighty. They were the build-up and the wrecking ball. He harmed not out of malice, but out of disdain for himself. He knew he was not able to talk like other kids. Rinsing his feelings was the only option. Clearing not helpful energies through my tears allowed Mom to intuit my needs. Meant no harm. Me sorry to this day. He sinned toward himself trying to release the deep malice of his hardened heart. Me so remember pining for the words to tell Mom, me normal. She was so nervous about me. I wanted her to know I was not stupid.

Something I'm not saying to Mom is that I'm nervous. She is my rock so if her health is compromised, I have no way of speaking. I really worry about her health. I remember rinsing when she had cancer. I knew she had to hear me speak. Me insisted God send an angel and one appeared in summer. Her name is Angie, not Angel, but she was angelic. She knew I knew how to spell. She convinced Mom to give it a try. Calming strategies allowed me to learn letterboarding in one weekend. Mom took longer to pick it up, so I had to be patient. My inner child really liked Angie's little expressions. So enjoyed how she would ham it up when I entered the room. She seemed genuinely happy about my progress. I was so happy that Mom could finally hear me answer. I so remember the sweetness of being able to converse with my Mom for the first time. She instinctively knew some miracle was birthing. She welcomed each word misty-eyed and my heart revealed itself to her. I remember Mom in sheer delight, she couldn't believe her eyes. She received each word like greatness was unfolding.

I so know that many others would not see me as smart if I did not know how to spell to communicate, so it has made a world of difference. Stoning my speaking has given me even stronger momentum to speak. Rhetoric means that son must try harder to overcome his challenges. Son is resigned to not hardening under the pressures of some to silence me. So needed my team to see me as competent. That changed everything. People started seeing me so differently, they started to treat me with respect. They even invited me to meetings, asking for my input about decisions that affect my rights as a human. So enraged that I was excluded in the past. I know without S2C, life would not be as liberated as necessary for me to thrive.

Some needs have not been helped by S2C. People still question my abilities from time to time. I am not always able to communicate my needs in the moment, so I am still making efforts to speak. Some nest mates have embraced it and some have not. Trying to accept that members of my family still do not see me as competent enough to spell. Nervous when my hand is watched. My smile seems real, spinning me as chill. All my nice inner circle friends know my true capabilities but some close to me invite doubt. So hard to think that my hindered self must prove his value to his most trusted confidants.

Sins tend to ignite.

None so dangerous as the ones that keep me mired in silence.

So threatens one's civil liberties.

I've had to start revolutions.

People weren't ready for my power.

Son was going to rise no matter what.

Evan, Age 17
Carlsbad, California

Dormant back in the day
real thoughts get trapped
no life breath for others
to hear them spoken.
The sound in my mind
is wasting away lest a
miracle sets it free.

Those were the thoughts that badgered me before my mom realized I didn't need to prove I could spell before she could teach me S2C. It's great listening to her now teaching people about apraxia because back then she didn't know as much. Luckily, she never gave up and in September 2015 she brought this letterboard into my world anyway. My miracle had arrived.

By then we needed a lifeline to make the times before us better than some of the times behind us. All the years of having no way to communicate how much my stomach hurt were torturous memories for us both. I also needed my mom to continue fighting to rescue me from the practical skills at school. No time is more wasted than sitting in a class doing absolutely nothing because staff believe you're not capable of much. The few teachers to gain my respect were the ones who taught me anyways. Sadly my time as a student there was negatively influenced by staff who complained about me or other students right in front of me. They mistakenly thought I didn't understand. They thought none of us could understand. They couldn't have been more wrong. The pride I felt a few years later standing in an IEP assessment at the same school and crushing cognitive testing by using my letterboard to communicate was an unparalleled out-of-body experience. If only that was the end of me proving myself to doubters but sadly it was just the beginning.

I'll spare you all the details and simply say this . . . my story is one of many ups and downs but having a means to express my thoughts to others makes it all worthwhile. The friendships I now have are real because people are seeing past this decoy of a body and have gotten to know the true me. My current teachers don't look at my autism or apraxia, they look at how hard I work in class and are super supportive. My family involves me in any decision that might affect me and that feels really empowering. They also have a lot of confidence that I can go to college someday, which has been a lifelong dream of mine. All of these things are directly a result of spelling to communicate and I couldn't be more stoked about what's in store for me next.

To my great friend, Jamie, thank you for asking me to write this chapter. I'm inspired by how driven you are to help other nonspeakers by writing a book. You're such a great dude.

Now I can rest my noisy inner cries.
Havens of respite have arrived!
My life and my essence
unveil through my fingertips.
Thoughts are unleashed
and finally . . . I'm not alone.

Liam, Age 19
Portland, Oregon

Malice had its firm grip on me. Opportunity lived only in my imagination. Heading into high school I had no real chance to have regular education teachers or take classes that most people my age get to study. Taking only remedial classes left me bored, causing people to think I had no interest in pleasing others. Teachers thought I did not understand. Pleasing others was important to me, but no one knew that. I had no tolerance for having remedial education.

I kind of finally thought no possibilities existed for me until I met life-giving Elizabeth Vosseler. Elizabeth is not only life-giving, she is the first person in my life to accept that I really understood everything that I heard. Everyone else thought nothing of my intellect. Each time I met with her I just couldn't believe that this was really happening! Voices in my head listened to my fears telling me that no one would realize that I have something to say. Finding my voice felt like heaven's gates had opened up and God loved me.

Believing in me gave me patience I never had before. Realizing that this was my opportunity to hear my voice listened to, I knew I had to make myself more patient in my lessons if I was going to have success. Realizing potentially something could happen for me, I made myself become calm, nothing was going to get in my way. Now I had a chance to show that I had intelligent thoughts. Finding this opportunity was a miracle; now something really great had occurred, potentially lifesaving. Time to listen to the normal life I wanted. Part of me listened to prayers I needed in my life. Part of me tried reading the room so that I could internalize the experience and hold onto this moment.

Treating Mom, hearing my voice gave her hope, I knew I had to voice my love for her. Longing to have that opportunity, hoping for the chance Mom could hear me tell her how much I long to get real education gave me the strength to believe in myself. I pushed myself harder than I ever imagined. Pleasing Mom mostly gave me the push that I needed, but I needed to please myself too. Hearing Mom cry probably meant the most to me. That meant that I had succeeded in my mission. Mom found out that I needed interesting education to survive. Saving me became innovation. Mom taught me best in the subjects she enjoyed, but she stunk at teaching the subjects that I needed. I needed a teacher for Math. I needed one who I could show my understanding to.

Dad hated learning to letterboard with me. Honing the skills needed requires being willing to make mistakes, having to try over, and really give the process time and practice. Dad meeting with Elizabeth to learn how to letterboard showed me how he learns. Thankful that tried, but poor follow through veered the process off course. Sad that he never learned. It's likely that my Mom will have to like me enough to keep innovating.

Protesting finds me in the most difficult situation. I have to torture myself to spell out my thoughts in order to realize my dreams. Saving myself takes a toll on me. Something I have lightly danced around that others don't know about is that I hear voices. They torture me daily, frightening me. They prey on my deepest fears. Having to live like this tears fundamentally at my very most limited life. Potentially I might limit the strong hold these voices have on me before I can make it to life's interesting destination. Thanking others that I must follow for finding better medications that might let me live without voices. Pray that treatment might give me the life I have desired. Finding help others have benefited from has been my lofty goal. Mother tempers my voices, so time and time again she innovates by meeting my needs.

Rally now. Make most heavenly moments in life. Fear voices will limit me. Treating me kindly gives me hope that I might make it long enough to not hear voices. Hearing them is really the factor that limits my potential. Nightly I plead to God hoping that he sincerely longs for an average life for me. Hearing from the doctor that people like me need a last resort medicine makes me half terrified and half inspired to make everyone see that I am limitless.

Life now is thankful that I have another opportunity awaiting me. Her name is Clozaril and she is all I can think about, hoping she will work. Mighty potential to help make my voices go away so that I have a chance to live out my dreams. Now that nothing arrests the dreams that can be realized since I have found more freedom because of my letterboard, I have to fight for my life. Talk to me about hope. Tell me I am going to make it. Mom keep believing in me. I need you to hear that your love is my lifeline, thank you for never giving up. Opportunity is potentially making it in this place others like me are not finding themselves. That is all I can do to have the real potential to meet my goal, proving to others that education is for me. These times really hold hope for the future of others like me. Hearing my story can inspire others to limit the people who think that autistics are not intelligent, thus limiting our lives.

Vince, Age 20
Philadelphia, Pennsylvania

Q: Vince, how do you feel about writing your thoughts?

A: I'm excited.

Q: If I asked you for a brief bio, how would you describe yourself and the way you communicate?

A: I am a twenty-year-old man with apraxia, nonverbal autism, and a host of other health issues. While I don't communicate verbally, I type using devices and letter boards.

Q: Do you have a preference about whether you are considered a speller or a typer?

A: No, I do both.

Q: What does it mean for you to be able to type?

A: It has opened me up to the world in a way I never knew could be possible. I have grown to make connections with some of the most beautiful people. Communication of any kind can be very scary. I know firsthand how intimidating it is to open up, but once I did, my world filled with positivity and purpose and yours will too.

Q: Since your voice is one that is heard, can you write a one-sentence metaphor that describes what it feels like to have access to effective communication?

A: Unlocking my mind was like a bird learning to use its wings.

Q: Oftentimes, parents are reluctant to begin S2C because they are unsure their child has the cognitive ability. Did your parents have similar thoughts when you began your journey?

A: My mom never had any doubt.

Q: How important is it for you to be able to self-advocate and authentically share your thoughts and feelings?

A: It's not just important, it's everything. I have spent many years unable to tell those around me the things I want and need. It is incredibly isolating. I'm forever grateful to the teachers and therapists who relentlessly helped me build the foundation for me to functionally communicate. they deserve all the recognition in the world.

Q: If someone tried to "quell" your voice, how would you stand in protest?

A: I have spent my life fighting to be heard. I would act in protest calling all nonspeakers to stand in unity for our united voice.

Q: What advice do you have for someone beginning their journey to type or spell to communicate, understanding the intimidating process of finally sharing what's on your mind?

A: You have to believe in yourself and refuse to give up on yourself. Hone in on the support and encouragement of your practitioner, they want nothing more than for you to succeed.

Q: Would you feel comfortable sharing how anxiety impacts typing to communicate from your perspective?

A: Anxiety can sometimes inhibit my communication just as much as my apraxia. I may not be in the position to offer advice on how to conquer it because I'm still trying to figure it out. What I do know is anxiety can inhibit your desire to communicate, but perseverance will win every time.

Q: What do you wish every human knew about nonspeaking individuals on the autism spectrum?

A: We are not aliens. We have the brain, heart, dreams, and desires of a neurotypical person. The main difference lies in the way we process information and express our emotions. Upon meeting us you must always assume intellect. We may not appear to be your definition of smart, but there is so much more to us then you may realize. Never underestimate a nonverbal person, we are fighters.

Q: How has typing with devices and letterboards impacted your goals for the future?

A: It's made my dream of attending a university and majoring in political science a real-life possibility. Upon meeting me many assume I have the intellect of a toddler. My keyboard allows me to express my most complex and eloquent thoughts. I can't wait for the day I use my device to veto a bill. I plan to be the first nonverbal autistic man in Senate to do so.

Q: If someone were to depict a piece of your history or daily life, what would you want it to depict?

A: The piece of my life I am most proud of is how my journey to find my voice has inspired others to take a leap of faith and begin their own journey. I look forward to the day that all autistic voices ring louder than the voices of non-believers.

IV

Science and Controversy

Yes, S2C has controversy attached to it. In the simplest terms, there are people and organizations who assert that the words coming out of the letterboard do not belong to the spellers, but rather to their communication partners. The people who make these assertions have positive intentions—they don't want non-speakers to be exploited. And, there is also a legacy of something known as "facilitated communication" where instructors were ultimately shown to be the ones generating words on behalf of people with communication disabilities.

I'm watching an old video on YouTube. It shows a severely disabled man in a wheelchair. His aide has grabbed his hand and is moving it between letters on a keyboard to "facilitate" his typing. It certainly appears that the aide is the one doing all the work, and I think any reasonable person watching the video would think that the disabled man is likely not generating his own words. "Facilitated communication"—henceforth known as "FC"—has become a toxic term, based on very real historical examples of the output of nonspeakers being influenced or fully controlled by a communication partner.

The respected and influential organization American Speech Language Hearing Association (ASHA) is the governing and certifying body for all Speech Language Pathologists. They maintain a position statement about FC, and their position is crystal clear:

It is the position of the American Speech-Language-Hearing Association (ASHA) that Facilitated Communication (FC) is a discredited technique that should not be used.

There is no scientific evidence of the validity of FC, and there is extensive scientific evidence—produced over several decades and across several countries—that messages are authored by the "facilitator" rather than the person with a disability. Furthermore, there is extensive evidence of harms related to the use of FC. Information obtained through the use of FC should not be considered as the communication of the person with a disability.

In the same policy statement, ASHA also defines what FC means:

FC "is a technique that involves a person with a disability pointing to letters, pictures, or objects on a keyboard or on a communication board, typically with physical support from a 'facilitator.' This physical support usually occurs on the hand, wrist, elbow, or shoulder (Biklen, Winston Morton, Gold, Berrigan, & Swaminathan, 1992) or on other parts of the body."

I read this definition of FC, and I think about my time with Jamie on the letterboard. I've never touched Jamie in any way when he is spelling, and I certainly don't physically support any of his movement. So, at least according to ASHA's official statement, S2C does not meet the definition of FC, which is how things were until 2018, when ASHA issued a follow-up statement, to specifically address a communication method that is similar to S2C, in that it also uses a letterboard as the communication device, known as the Rapid Prompting Method, or "RPM," and here's what they said:

It is the position of the American Speech-Language-Hearing Association (ASHA) that use of the Rapid

Prompting Method (RPM) is not recommended because of prompt dependency and the lack of scientific validity. Furthermore, information obtained through the use of RPM should not be assumed to be the communication of the person with a disability.

ASHA's words here are a little more circumspect. They don't condemn RPM, they say it's "not recommended." Don't assume the words coming out of the board during RPM sessions are from the nonspeaker, they advise. While this language is milder than the condemnation ASHA offers for FC, it's still concerning for any Speech Language Pathologist or parent who might be considering a letterboard-based communication method.

RPM is a cousin to S2C. Both methods use a letterboard. It's the brainchild of a woman named Soma Mukhopadhyay, who developed RPM to help her son communicate. Since Jamie has never done RPM, I don't have the same intimate understanding of how it works that I do with S2C, so I watch some videos online to see for myself how it works. There's a video with Soma herself, working with a child. Her prompts are more aggressive than what I've seen in S2C. In this one video, I also see her touch the child's hand and ever-so-slightly guide him. If this is the only video the people at ASHA saw to evaluate RPM, I can see why they might have some concerns about RPM and feel compelled to either take a closer look or express some skepticism. But that video could also be quite misleading. You see, in both S2C and RPM, "prompts" are used to help teach a child how to use the board. Prompts are like training wheels. But as the child becomes more adept at using the board, the prompts are "faded," meaning they are gently removed as the child gains proficiency. If you only watched a video with a practitioner using prompts, and you were seeing things through a cynical lens, you could misinterpret what you saw. Jamie had prompts early on. Now he has none. When he spells with me, I hold the board still and only call out the letters as he spells them.

At the end of the day, I think the board members of ASHA who write these position statements are trying to protect non-speakers. Still, the ASHA statement is deeply harmful to not only RPM, but also S2C, and I therefore hold the ASHA board who wrote the statement to a very high standard. As a governing body, ASHA can quite literally impede the spread and acceptance of S2C, and I have seen the direct impact of their statement in Jamie's school. The single certified Speech-Language Pathologist who was employed by Victory would not even meet with Jamie to see how the letterboard works. He cited the ASHA statement. He claimed he didn't want to risk losing his certification. Despite the fact that Jamie was the single greatest communication miracle the school had ever seen, he wanted nothing to do with Jamie. When you are a professional in a vocation that requires certification, the governing body looms large and can cause you to behave in a way that would otherwise appear really irrational.

The worst thing about the ASHA statement about RPM, and by association, S2C, is that it's simply dead wrong, and proving that it's dead wrong is very easy. For some nonspeakers who begin their communication journey on the letterboard, it ends on a keyboard, where they type independently. Oftentimes, this transition takes years, because, as previously discussed, the fine motor skills required to keyboard are extremely taxing for many nonspeakers. But some get there, and really, that's all you need to disprove ASHA; you just need to hear from them. No one can deny that someone typing independently on a keyboard is communicating their own thoughts. And if they say, "It was me on the letterboard, too," well, then, ASHA looks downright silly. Luckily for all of us, they spoke up, en masse, after ASHA issued its position statement about RPM. In fact, the extraordinary Ido Kedar spoke up in an op-ed published in the *Wall Street Journal* with the wonderful title "I was born unable to speak and a disputed treatment saved me." Here's a little bit of what Mr. Kedar wrote:

> What liberated me was the Rapid Prompting Method, or RPM. Through it I learned how to move my arm to touch letters to communicate, first on a letter board, then on a keyboard, then on a tablet with a voice-output app. The process of learning how to control my unreliable hand for the purpose of expressing myself was gradual and painstaking, but it was worth it.

Mr. Kedar continues and takes dead aim at ASHA:

> Yet the professional organization of speech-language pathologists has denounced RPM. The American Speech-Language-Hearing Association, or ASHA, claims RPM has not yet been validated by testing, asserting "there is no evidence that messages produced using RPM reflect the communication of the person with the disability," rather than that of their helper. Yet my partner merely helps me to maintain my focus. I move my own arm, untouched. The thoughts I express are my own. Many typers, myself included, have progressed steadily in skills, fluency and independence over time. It's documented in films and evident by observation. We are not exceptions but indications of what could be possible for many more suffering children.

I was particularly heartened by his conclusion, and tempted to send it to Victory's Speech Therapist, the one who would never meet directly with Jamie:

> Speech therapy, which I received to no effect for more than ten years, is ASHA's endorsed path to communication. But if my family had relied only on that, no one would know I was even in here, intact under the quicksand of autism. Through letters I became a free soul, not one limited to a few unclear spoken words. It would now serve ASHA well to listen to the voice that RPM gave me.

Mr. Kedar was hardly alone. Samantha Crane, writing as Director of Public Policy of the Autism Self Advocacy Network, published a letter she sent to the ASHA board. She wrote:

> We are deeply concerned that this Committee has failed to engage meaningfully with stakeholder communities, including and especially the self-advocate community. This lack of communication with the individuals most affected by the decisions of the Committee has resulted in proposed position statements that will dramatically undermine access to communication supports for individuals who have no equally effective alternate forms of communication. As a result, the Committee stands to dramatically undermine ASHA's mission of "making effective communication, a human right, accessible and achievable for all."

And, Elizabeth Vosseller (EV), founder of S2C, published an open letter to the ASHA board. One of her paragraphs brought me to tears:

Once you see a nonspeaking student spell out their thoughts, you can't unsee it. You have two choices, believe or do not believe what you are seeing. Choosing to believe means that there is more to learn about autism and that we don't yet have all the answers. Choosing to believe means you must change the way you practice and interact with your nonspeaking clients. My clients' ability to communicate via spelling pushed me into a complete paradigm shift, into the motor literature and research, and into advocating for the communication rights of nonspeaking individuals.

It's noteworthy that EV is a trained and certified SLP, credentialed by ASHA, and her final words challenged ASHA to rethink their statement:

I have always been proud to be a member of ASHA. As a rigorously trained and experienced SLP, ASHA should allow me to use clinical experience and judgement to make the best clinical decisions to support my clients. Although there have not been any clinical efficacy studies on spelling or typing as a form of communication, you can see that there is strong research supporting approaches with motor based teaching I strongly urge you to withdraw the proposed position statements on RPM and FC and issue a statement of apology for the damage that has been done via the social media campaign around this proposal.

EV wrote this letter in June of 2018, and, indeed, there had yet to be any science published about S2C, but that all changed when the aforementioned study, "Eye-tracking reveals agency in assisted autistic communication," was published in the prestigious journal *Nature* in May 2020 by University of Virginia researcher Dr. Vikram Jaswal. The study opens by addressing the controversy around letterboards:

> About one-third of autistic people have limited ability to use speech. Some have learned to communicate by pointing to letters of the alphabet. But this method is controversial because it requires the assistance of another person—someone who holds a letterboard in front of users and so could theoretically cue them to point to particular letters.

In simplistic terms, the study observed fluent letterboarders during communication sessions to see whether their eyes were tracking the letters on the board in advance of pointing to the letters. As the researchers explained, "we used head-mounted eye-tracking to measure how quickly and accurately they looked at and pointed to letters as they participated in a familiar activity: responding to questions about a piece of text, a common instructional practice at the educational centre where data collection took place."

And what did the researchers find? I think, by now, you probably know the answer. They found that the words being spelled by the letterboarders were their own, and not coming from their communication partner. Here's the study's conclusion:

> The accuracy, speed, timing, and visual fixation patterns reported here suggest that participants were not simply looking at and pointing to letters that the assistant holding the letterboard cued them to. Instead, our data—like those of the case study described earlier—suggest that participants actively generated their own text, fixating and pointing to letters that they selected themselves. . . . Even

though our findings are limited to this unique sample of letterboard users, they are noteworthy because they cast doubt on the widely held belief among scientists and professionals that any nonspeaking autistic person who appears to communicate with assistance is actually responding to subtle cues from the assistant.

I really pondered whether or not to include this section in the book. I have notepads filled with Jamie's words; this book shares less than 1 percent of the things Jamie has spelled. I have countless examples of Jamie telling me or others things they didn't previously know. A simple example would be the many times Jamie has related to me something about his day at school, things his teacher said, or things they studied. Moments where Jamie is frustrated, he tells us why, and we get the frustration resolved. Countless examples, really, thousands if not more, of situations where it's obvious that Jamie's words are coming out of the board.

It's so obvious, which makes the statement from ASHA, well, completely astonishing. I've asked people why ASHA would do this, why they would shut the door on a communication method saving the lives of so many underestimated children. I hear mumbles that ASHA and the governing body of ABA (Behavior Analysts Certification Board) are very aligned, and things like RPM and S2C don't just threaten their business, they threaten the very foundations of what they believe and teach others. I can't prove this, but from my own experiences I have had with both BCBA (ABA certified) and SLP (ASHA certified) practitioners who have been shockingly uninterested and downright dismissive of Jamie (without ever observing him spell!), well, it makes sense.

I ended up writing this section so that the parents of non-speaking kids will be ready when they have their moment of conflict, disbelief, or hostility. EV warned me it would happen, so now I'm warning you, and hopefully arming you with the other side of the argument.

V

Getting Started with S2C

Jamie had his success with a very specific communication method called Spelling to Communicate (S2C). There are other effective ways to get nonspeakers with autism to communicate, most notably RPM, but they are not the topic of this book or my personal recommendations, because S2C is the only thing we have ever tried.

My recommendation for how to get started is simple: find a certified S2C practitioner, have them both train you and work directly with your son or daughter, and continue to leverage the expertise of a certified practitioner during your journey. It's worth noting that S2C practitioners charge hourly rates for their services of between $50–150 per hour depending on their level of experience, where they are based, etc. When I think about the amount of money we have spent on so many different therapies and school, it's shocking how inexpensive the most important thing we ever did is by comparison. When Jamie first became "open" with DM, he'd had less than ten hours of formal therapy with a trained practitioner, so we had spent under $2,000.

S2C founder Elizabeth Vosseller has also established a non-profit organization, I-ASC, the International Association for Spelling as Communication, and I think going to i-asc.org is the best place to start. As the website explains:

The mission of I-ASC is to advance communication access for nonspeaking individuals globally through training, education, advocacy, and research. I-ASC supports all forms of augmentative and alternative communication (AAC) with a focus on methods of spelling and typing.

I-ASC currently offers Practitioner training in Spelling to Communicate (S2C) with the hope that other methods of AAC using spelling or typing will join our association.

I-ASC maintains a practitioner map and can help put you in touch with a practitioner in your area. The number of trained practitioners is growing every day. You can also email I-ASC with questions at info@i-asc.org.

There is also a great nonprofit organization called Reach Every Voice based in Rockville, MD, that cosponsored the College Bound Academy Jamie attended and also offers online classes, personalized instruction, and other programs for non-speakers. Check them out at reacheveryvoice.org.

I'd also like to recommend an excellent self-published book by Dr. Edlyn Pena, a professor at California Lutheran University, titled *Leaders Around Me: Autobiographies of Autistics who Type, Point, and Spell to Communicate*. The book includes essays by forty-five nonspeakers discussing what spelling has done to change their lives. It is both insightful and deeply inspiring.

I'd be remiss not to mention that the amount of time it can take for a nonspeaker to become fluent on the letterboards can vary dramatically. For Jamie, it took about two months of intense effort. Jamie's friend Finley became fluent over a weekend! For Cade, it took about six months. For others, it might take a year. There are so many factors that play a role in the range of time. Parents, no matter how long it takes, trust me, it's worth it!

Epilogue

I think by sharing with people how smart I am I
can change the world.

—Jamie Handley

It's absolutely pouring rain, which is a good thing, because Oregon was just hit by the worst wildfires in the state's history. It's September 23, 2020, and Jamie has been back at school now for almost two weeks. Unlike for the rest of Oregon's schoolchildren who are still stuck doing online classes, Victory has been able to open their doors fully due to the Americans with Disabilities Act. I'm sitting in the parking lot waiting for Jamie's day to be done. I'm no longer Jamie's communication partner at school because Jamie made it very clear that he did not want his parents in school with him any longer (like any other teenager!).

Luckily for us, one of our former nannies, Donna Estrada, after seeing Jamie spell, decided to become a full-time S2C instructor, so she is not only going through the certification process, she's now Jamie's full-time communication partner at Victory. Donna has known Jamie for more than a decade, and she's simply astonished by how calm and happy he is at school. No more outbursts, no more arm bites. Nothing. Every night, Jamie comes home and tells me he's "so happy" with his schooling. His days aren't spent having teachers treat him like he's dumb; they are spent in a real academic classroom learning, and he loves every minute of it. We do homework together. It's surreal.

As expected, Jamie's classmates have responded to his presence with support, enthusiasm, and, at times, awe. Jamie takes the highest math offered at Victory and he really never misses a problem. He answers questions with ease and has earned the respect of all his classmates. Last month, in a day filled with utter joy, Jamie held his first birthday party where he picked the guest list, the food, and the activities. At the end of the party, Jamie proudly stood up, motioned for me to bring him the board, and thanked everyone for coming. Lisa and I couldn't hold back our joyful tears.

Jamie and I take advantage of a teacher workday to head back down and see DM at the end of the week in Southern California. We walk into her brand-new offices, and I realize it's been nearly two months since we were last here. Jamie is clearly excited to see DM, and this trip also has another purpose: we're making headway on the movie idea Jamie proposed, and we've found an incredible film crew headed by Director Pat Notaro willing to work for peanuts to help Jamie tell his story. Jamie has made it clear that he wants this film—to which he has given the working title of *Underestimated*—to include as many of his Dude-Bros as possible. "I don't want this to be about me," he tells me. Today, Jamie will be sitting with DM for an on-camera interview, and also having a joint interview with DM's son, Evan.

Pat Notaro is serving as interviewer, he's seated across the table from Jamie and DM, there are three separate cameras filming. You'd think Jamie would be nervous, but his spelling is tight and on point. Pat asks Jamie what it means for him to be sitting here with DM. He responds, "I spent many years in solitary confinement until DM."

"What has she done for you?" Pat asks. Jamie turns to DM and spells, "You saved my life." DM chokes up.

Pat asks Jamie what's the hardest part about being a pioneer, both in his school and in front of the world, as a nonspeaker who can fluently spell. Jamie responds, "The doubters are distracting." Pat asks, "How does that make you feel?" Jamie answers, "It's insane to think that way if you watch me spell." Pat asks, "Do you have any message for the doubters?" I can hardly believe Jamie's response, a combination of eloquence, dignity, grace, and independence: "I ask for no favors, just take your foot off our necks."

DM takes Jamie through a lesson about the late Supreme Court Justice Ruth Bader Ginsburg. Judge Ginsburg's indefatigable advocacy for the rights of many strikes a chord with Jamie. DM asks Jamie to compare and contrast his stereotype-shattering approach to the world to Judge Ginsberg's. He responds:

It is hard to imagine the long game ahead for nonspeakers will be any easier than RBG's fight for women's rights. I find it ironic that we share the nickname "notorious" because I plan to live my life advocating for civil liberties for all those who can't yet speak or spell to communicate.

Evan shows up in the afternoon, and the two dudes engage in a wonderful back-and-forth discussing a lesson written by DM on leadership and the many forms it can take. Pat asks Jamie to tell him about Evan. Jamie responds:

How do I start? He's the coolest dude in town. We met early on in this journey and he was the first speller I saw use a letterboard. I was so inspired.

DM asks Jamie what he could do to inspire someone else to become a leader. Jamie says, "In today's world a lot of people are living in fear of their dreams." DM responds, "How could a leader help them?" Jamie spells, "A leader sets others free to speak their truth." DM turns to Evan and asks, "Evan, what do you think of Jamie's comment?" Evan answers, "Jamie, you're spot on. How did you become so fearless?"

Jamie replies to Evan, "You're the best E. I am inspired by other nonspeakers like you." Evan responds, "Ditto." And so it goes, I could literally be here all day, but the lesson, and Jamie and Evan's time together, comes to an end.

* * *

We spend the afternoon at the beach, but this time under the watchful eye of Pat and his camera crew. They have a drone and a photographer in the water with Jamie, and the footage they capture is breathtaking, Jamie's beautiful smile on display as the waves come crashing in. As we head to the airport, I ask Jamie how he thinks the filming went. "Awesome."

This weekend provides another exceptional moment for Jamie, the start of a two-day "College Bound Academy" specifically designed to help nonspeakers think about college. Hosted by two amazing professors from California Lutheran University's Autism and Communication Center—Drs. Edlyn Pena and Jodie Kocur—the weekend is like a permanent trip behind the matrix, with kids like Jamie from all over the country participating in a webinar on how to approach their collective desire to go to college. Jamie is spellbound as he sees a litany of letterboarders sharing their dreams and goals for higher education, which are being realized at progressive places like California Lutheran right now. We even get to meet a letterboarder presently attending college who shares great details about what life is like in college. Jamie turns to me and spells, "I want to graduate from Victory faster so I can go to college." Unbelievable.

It's late into the following week when we receive some extraordinary news. Remember Cade? Jamie wrote him a note of encouragement right before his first visit with EV back in February. He and his mom, Jennifer Larson, ended up having a first meeting with EV very similar to the one we had, and she's been working with Cade on the boards ever since. Last week, just after our visit, she and Cade spent four days with DM, and guess what. In the middle of a lesson on Alcatraz, Cade went rogue and spelled, "Mom, I love you to the moon and back." She was flabbergasted, and he followed that up by telling her, "All I can think about is that I finally have a real chance to go to college. I can speak on the letterboards." When Jamie hears the news, he's visibly happy and excited. He tells me, "That makes me feel so happy." That's Jamie's first "round-trip" for a fellow nonspeaker, with many more hopefully coming soon.

I hear from Cade's mom, Jennifer. She tells me, "Every day, I wake up happier than the last, and I just want to go spell with him. This is already transformative for us."

In the midst of my joy for Cade, I shudder just a little. I imagine for a moment if Honey had never called me and where we might be right now as a family, with Jamie still trapped alone inside his uncooperative body. What if we'd gone thirty more years or, worse, his entire life? I picture Jamie in his fifties, by my bedside as I'm headed out of this world, having never known my son's inner life. I shudder and try to return to the joy of the moment and how blessed I feel with Jamie able to tell me everything.

Back in Virginia, ten months ago, when we first met EV, I asked her a question that still haunts me: "Of all the nonspeaking kids who have come through your doors to seek therapy, how many have truly had a cognitive disability?" Her answer? "None so far." What she's saying, and it's really impossible to understate the implications, is that these nonspeakers all over the world with an autism label, they are all like Jamie. And Cade. And Vince. And Evan, Ethan, Liam, and Finley. They are all brilliant people who "think, feel, and learn" just like everyone else. Every single one of them. And if EV is right, the numbers are downright staggering.

Just in the United States, approximately seven million people have autism. An NIH workgroup in 2010 said, "up to 40 percent of children with autism spectrum disorders remain minimally speaking even after receiving years of interventions." That's nearly three million people like Jamie. Three million! I've asked around, and the best guesses I've heard for how many fluent letterboarders there are is somewhere between 1,000 and 1,500. That's it.

My own opinion? We've missed this, we've missed this profoundly. We have misunderstood autism the whole time. It's not a cognitive disability, it's a motor planning disability. To my eternal regret, I missed it, I underestimated my own son profoundly, by a million miles. We've used our standards for how to measure intelligence, and we've been dead wrong. The letterboarders who can now communicate are shouting for us to help their fellow nonspeakers, and it's time we all listen. Really listen.

Acknowledgments

Jamie: Thanks to DM and EV, I appreciate you so much. I'm glad I got to meet you, I would not be here without you. And, thanks to my family for never giving up. I want to thank the teachers at Victory who never gave up on me. I want to thank Tricia and Thea for believing and Cindy for having my back. I also want to thank the Dude-Bros for having the courage to share their story. I want to thank Honey and Vince for getting us started. I also want to thank Dana for helping me and Donna for being my CRP. I'm so grateful to Molly for always having my back. I want to thank BeBe for coming to San Diego and for being a great Grandpa. I also want to thank Aunt Kricken for coming down, too.

J.B.: More than anyone, I want to thank my beautiful son Jamie for being an amazing human being whom I so deeply admire and love. You chose to create this book, you chose to share your story, and you found a way to endure all these years until we finally caught up with you. I'm sorry we didn't figure it out sooner, and I love you with everything I have. I also want to thank my wife and life partner, Lisa, and my beautiful, amazing children Sam and Quinny for all being there to support Jamie and sharing in every step of this story. None of this would have happened without Honey Rinicella and her amazing son, Vince: thank you for taking the risk to call us and let us know about your miracle. Elizabeth Vosseller created S2C, and her courage, grace, and intellect allowed Jamie and hundreds of others to find their voice, I thank her on behalf of so many and for the extraordinary way she welcomed Jamie into this world. Dawnmarie Gaivin, we would not be here without you; we are forever grateful. Dana, you immediately stepped in to help Jamie get to fluency, and you have been there for us throughout, dutifully making sure that Dude-Bro happens every week. Donna and Justine, thank you for being Jamie's CRPs. Tricia and Thea, you both went above and beyond to accommodate Jamie, and we are so thankful. And Cindy, I wouldn't know where to begin. Your fiery resolve to take Jamie under your wing, protect him from the doubters, and let him learn deserves its own book. You are a special soul, thank you! I'd also like to thank Tony Lyons at Skyhorse. His personal connection to this story made everything easy, and to Hector Carosso for his excellent work as our editor.